Your Child's Teeth

Your Child's Teeth

A PARENT'S GUIDE TO MAKING
AND KEEPING THEM PERFECT

Stephen J. Moss

D.D.S.

*Illustrated with
drawings and photographs*

Houghton Mifflin Company Boston

Library of Congress Cataloging in Publication Data

Moss, Stephen J.
   Your child's teeth.
   Includes index.
    1. Teeth—Care and hygiene. 2. Children—
Dental care. I. Title. [DNLM: 1. Oral health—
Popular works. 2. Pedodontics—Popular works.
3. Preventive dentistry—In infancy and childhood—
Popular works.   WU113 M913y]
RK61.M87   617.6'01   77-5691
ISBN 0-395-25344-6
ISBN 0-395-27592-x (pbk.)

Printed in the United States of America

M 12 11 10 9 8 7 6 5 4 3

To my dear wife, Lydia, who proved these concepts to be true by helping me to start our sons on the road toward a goal that neither she nor I ever reached — healthy, perfect, lifetime teeth.

"Little can be accomplished for grown-up people; the intelligent man begins with the child."

— *Goethe,* 1776

"Goodnight Mommy; Goodnight Daddy. I'm going to brush my teeth and go to bed."

— *Jonathan Moss,* 1976

"Just as the twig is bent, the tree's inclined."

— *Alexander Pope,* 1734

"I'll take a carrot stick instead; it won't make holes in my teeth."

— *David Moss,* 1977

Contents

Introduction

Part One of *Your Child's Teeth* is the heart of the book, for it covers your child's earliest years, the years before the dentist is consulted on how to care for the child's teeth. The most important time in your child's dental history is not the day he meets the dentist for the first time. It's long, long before that.

Beginning with your baby before birth, and covering the period from conception to first tooth, and later the period from first tooth to adult tooth, the topics discussed make up a directory of the information you'll need to guide you and your children through the early years of preventive dental care.

The most important time for teeth is when no one is actually thinking about them.

The message in this book is not subliminal. It's spelled out very clearly.

We can break the chain of tooth decay.

It's as simple — and as profound — as that.

Today, dental disease is totally preventable. It can be accomplished in one generation. If you decide that it's worthwhile to raise children who have strong, clean, straight teeth, no cavities, no pain, no dental disease, and better health all around, you can do it. As John and Yoko told us, "The war is over. If you want it."

This means that bad teeth don't "run in the family." There is just no hereditary excuse for cavities or for crooked teeth. What we do pass down from generation to generation are eating habits, muscular patterns, attitudes toward oral cleanliness, and so forth. If your grandmother had a history of dental problems, it was because neither she nor her parents knew how to take care of her teeth. If your grandfather wore dentures, it may be because he lived at a time when teeth were pulled to "cure" all kinds of ailments, from rheumatism to poor eyesight. If you yourself grew up with memories of cavities, gum problems, crooked teeth, and scary visits to a dentist, this book may be unsettling — even unbelievable — and frustrating for you to read. But your own child has been born in the age of prevention, and if he has eight cavities in his teeth by the time he's five years old, it will be because somebody has failed to do something.

It's not easy to change deep-seated behavior patterns. It takes a revolution in your lifestyle; it takes the determination to do things differently from the way your parents and friends and neighbors do things. Any such basic change in the way people live their lives is radical.

Suppose we suggest to a young mother (because she's the one who is usually around at mealtimes) that cleaning her baby's mouth should begin soon before the child's teeth come into his or her mouth.

The young mother hesitates. None of her friends do this; her mother didn't do this. Besides, she is unfamiliar with the interior of her baby's mouth and is reluctant to reach inside. She thinks she is going to introduce some infection (although just the opposite is true). Can she overcome this acculturated attitude? Getting into the habit of cleaning the child's mouth twice a day — from the time the baby is about nine months old, first with a gauze pad and later with a soft toothbrush — is one of the foundations of preventive dentistry. It is up to Mom or Dad to do this until the child is old enough — about five years — to take over by himself. Such behavior on the parent's part is going to require dedication and a cultural change.

There have been a number of new developments in the science of dentistry, particularly in the science of dentistry *for children.* We have reached the time when dental caries is as preventable as polio, mumps, or diphtheria. In fact, a child can go from birth to a full complement of adult teeth without a bad dental experience, without decay, and often without crooked teeth.

Clinical experiments have expanded knowledge in dentistry. While it was suspected for a long time that there were three links in the chain of tooth decay — sugar-containing foods, bacteria, and a susceptible tooth — it is only recently that laboratory experiments have clearly proved the connection between these factors and decay. This clinical knowledge calls for a three-way effort to break the chain, through new approaches to diet, to oral hygiene, and to strengthening the resistance of teeth to decay.

New developments in psychology lead many psychologists to believe that personality is developed by the time the baby is eighteen months (some put it even earlier). Although we've said that bad teeth are not inherited, we do know that a cultural disposition toward food is set very early in life. By the time the child is eighteen months old, we may, as parents, have already set his lifetime predilection for certain foods, as well as the way he chews what he eats. Gum pads make perfectly adequate chewing surfaces. A child who chews vigorously is working the muscles of his jaw even before his teeth come in, and as a result will develop his jaw muscles and his salivary glands.

One parent will decide to breast-feed; another will opt for bottle-feeding. One parent may feed a child soft foods, thinking them more digestible or fearing that the child may aspirate more solid fare or choke on it. Another parent, less anxious, will let her child chew on carrot sticks or celery or crusty toast. When my own children were quite young, I let them put in their mouths any food they could pick up and aim correctly. We now know that a child who chews and works his jaws is strengthening his oral-facial muscles and establishing his neuromuscular pathways. Here I shall discuss the physical nature of the food itself — its texture — not its nutritional value. (I'll cover both aspects in Chapter 5, "Diet Decisions.")

The clinical significance of recent laboratory findings has, of course, had an impact on the dental profession. Dentists now know that it is possible for a child to grow to adulthood with strong teeth that will last a lifetime. Parents, dentists, and children must become allies, each motivating and supporting the other. New findings in persuasive prevention — otherwise known as the carrot and the stick

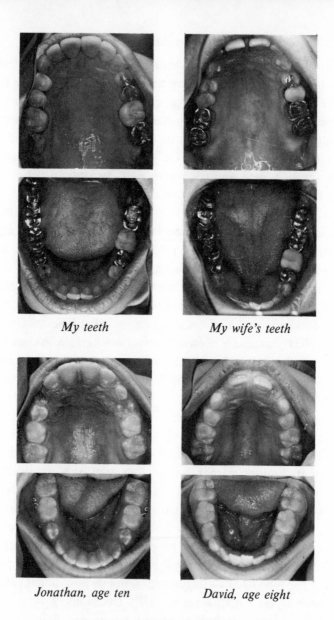

My teeth　　　*My wife's teeth*

Jonathan, age ten　　　*David, age eight*

MY FAMILY ALBUM:
HOW DEFENSIVE DENTISTRY WORKS

Both my wife and I have had many cavities. We have spent hours having them repaired. We must have imparted some susceptibility to our two sons. Yet by practicing defensive dentistry in our home we have overcome the children's susceptibility to cavities. As you can see from the photographs, we have given them perfect teeth. You can do this for your children.

— will be discussed. Most dentists are ready to change their old image, and concentrate on preventing disease rather than repairing its results.

Look at the photographs, opposite, of the parents and children in my own family. Both my wife and I have experienced a sad history of dental decay, despite the facts that my father was a dentist and that my wife's family could have afforded the best dental care available. We decided to try defensive dentistry before the birth of our first child. Now our children, Jonathan, eleven years old, and David, nine, are free of dental disease. Our "family album" shows it — bad teeth are not inherited. Cavities don't just happen.

The fact that it works in my own family leads me to believe that preventive dentistry can work. Otherwise, I would not urge you to follow a course of action you might find strange or difficult. Of course, because I am a dentist, the orientation in my house is a little different. My wife, for instance, is sure that I will turn into a raging beast if a cavity is discovered in our children's teeth. That's why, on a typical morning, with breakfast on the stove, the phone ringing, the search for socks and books and pencils in full swing, and the school bus honking at the front door, she'll oversee the tooth-brushing detail.

PART I

A PRIMER ON
YOUR CHILD'S TEETH

From Conception to First Tooth

THE DEVELOPING TOOTH

About three months after conception, as the growing baby graduates from embryo to fetus, the teeth are already beginning to form and to be recognizable. Which teeth form before birth? Some parts of all of the twenty primary teeth. (Primary teeth also go by the names *baby teeth, milk teeth,* and *first teeth.*) Except for a tiny piece of the first permanent molar, the rest of the permanent teeth wait until right after birth to start forming.

If the baby is going to be a thumb-sucker, chances are she already has the habit well underway by the seventh month in the uterus. (Knowing that today most dentists and doctors believe that thumb-suckers are born, not made, may help you to relax later.) In the weeks before birth, the baby is already making sucking and chewing movements with her jaws, in preparation for nursing. In short, even before birth, the mouth is getting ready for its complex tasks.

A nutritious, balanced diet is good for anyone, anytime . . . but for an expectant mother, it pays double benefits by contributing to the health of both mother and child. However, while it's all to the good to eat a balanced diet and to stay well and avoid harmful drugs, there is really not much a mother-to-be can do to affect her baby's teeth *directly.* Most of what goes on in the embryonic stages takes place automatically. The minerals that are needed to form a baby's developing teeth are taken from her mother's bloodstream, and unless she is actually undernourished, nothing will interfere with the

---

Chronology of the Development of a Tooth

Although the first teeth will not make their appearance in the baby's mouth until about six months after birth, the manufacture of a tooth begins as early as the seventh week of pregnancy. This is the developmental pattern:

- tooth-bud formation,
- beginning of crown formation,
- completion of crown,
- beginning of root formation,
- eruption of tooth into mouth,
- completion of root formation.

---

ability of the baby's tooth-forming cells to turn these basic salts into normal dentin and enamel cells.

If a child is going to get cavities in his first set of teeth, it will probably be in one of two areas: the biting surfaces of the molars, or between the molars, where there is proximal contact.

Why talk about this now? Because now — before birth — is when the top surfaces and the side surfaces of the molar teeth are beginning to form. How resistant these caries-sensitive surfaces will be depends on how well these teeth mineralize. The mother, by balancing the necessary calcium and phosphorus and vitamins in her bloodstream, contributes to this successful hardening.

We know that fluoride is a great help to developing teeth, but not very much fluoride crosses the placental barrier. Because there is no way to get more fluoride into an unborn baby's teeth through the mother's diet, strengthening the teeth with fluoride will have to wait until later.

There are three things that may happen to the expectant mother that could directly affect her baby's teeth.

If she gets a fever from a virus or some other infection (a common occurrence between the fifth and ninth months of pregnancy), the delicate balance of calcium and phosphorous salts in her bloodstream could be upset. This would affect the quality and quantity of tooth structure that is forming in the fetus. The disruption will continue for as long as it takes the mother's system to regain its balance.

If her physician gives her an antibiotic containing tetracycline, the matrix of the developing fetal teeth might become stained. Later, when the teeth come into the mouth, they will be discolored. The color may range from dark gray through yellow to bright orange, depending on how much tetracycline the mother gets, how long she takes it, and at what time during pregnancy. Most physicians don't prescribe tetracycline for pregnant mothers; its use is becoming rare. A woman who is pregnant but doesn't yet "show" should tell the doctor that she's expecting.

If the expectant mother gives birth before term, it is possible that the child's teeth will be affected. There is some evidence today that full-term children have fewer cavities. This is because those areas of the teeth that are mineralizing just around the time of birth are the ones most susceptible to decay.

WHAT TO DO BEFORE THE BABY COMES: EAT RIGHT*

For nine months before his birth, the baby depends entirely on his mother for nourishment. This nourishment comes from two sources: the food the mother eats and the tissues of her body. The calcium, phosphorus, and vitamins needed for good teeth and bones, for instance, can be supplied in a balanced diet that contains four basic food groups: the milk group, the meat and fish group, the fruit and vegetable group, and the enriched or whole-grain cereal and bread group.

There are many ways of selecting and preparing the important foods. The menus suggested here are just *one* selection. They show how the basic diet of a normal, healthy woman can be added to during pregnancy and nursing.

*Adapted from *What to Eat,* published by the National Dairy Council.

Healthy Active Woman	*Pregnant Woman*	*Nursing Mother*
BREAKFAST		
Citrus fruit, melon, or tomato juice	Citrus fruit, melon, or tomato juice	Citrus fruit, melon, or tomato juice
Cereal with milk or egg	Cereal with milk or egg	Cereal with milk or egg
Buttered toast	Buttered toast	Buttered toast
MIDMORNING		
	Milk	Milk
LUNCH		
Creamed vegetable soup	Creamed vegetable soup	Creamed vegetable soup
Cottage cheese salad with fruits or vegetables	Cottage cheese, meat, or egg salad	Lean meat or cottage cheese
Bread and butter	Bread and butter	Potato
Fruit pie	Fruit	Vegetable salad
Milk		Bread and butter
		Fruit pie
		Milk
MIDAFTERNOON		
	Milk	Milk
DINNER		
Meat	Tomato juice	Tomato juice
Potato	Lean meat	Lean meat
Vegetable	Potato	Potato
Cake or ice cream	Vegetable, green or yellow	Vegetable, green or yellow
	Ice cream	Bread and butter
	Milk	Ice cream with fruit
		Milk
BEDTIME		
Milk	Milk	Milk

Use whole milk, or substitute skim milk as part of the daily milk intake to reduce calories.

All cereals and bread should be enriched or whole grain.

Eat as wide a variety of fruits and vegetables as possible.

Use cheese or more eggs sometimes in place of meat, fish or poultry; also use dried beans or split peas, as in bean or pea soup.

Because of their rich supply of minerals and vitamins, liver, kidney, or heart should often be included. If you take a vitamin-mineral supplement, regard it as *insurance,* not as a substitute for good nutrition. Check with your obstetrician on questions of nutrition, diet, and weight.

Old Wives' Tale

"The baby took all the calcium from my teeth!"

If the mother has sufficient calcium in her diet, there's no problem. If her diet is deficient in calcium, the calcium requirements of the embryo will be met first, and some of the calcium may come from the mother's bones; it will not come from her teeth.

There are hormonal changes during pregnancy, and one of the results of these changes is swelling of the gums. Swollen gums harbor food debris and bacteria; gum disease and decay may develop. You might blame your toothache on pregnancy, but don't blame your baby. Just be especially careful. Brush. Floss. Get a thorough cleaning from a dentist . . . but avoid x-rays if possible.

THE NEW BABY

At birth, health care starts with a thorough examination by the obstetrician and the pediatrician. Any congenital abnormalities in the dentition, such as a harelip or a cleft palate, should be diagnosed by these doctors and the baby referred for proper treatment. But remember that unusual and rare conditions are just that — unusual and rare. Your baby will probably have the good start in life that every parent hopes his child will have. If there is a problem, my advice is that the parent resist surgery for as long as possible, unless the problem interferes with the baby's ability to eat and survive. It's tough on the parents psychologically, but the older the child is, the bigger the parts that the surgeon will have to work with — and the final result will be better for the child.

Sometimes, shortly after birth, parents or physicians notice little white spots on the upper palate (the roof of the mouth). These are little keratinized structures called "Epstein's pearls." (Keratin is a tough, fibrous protein found in nails, hair, and teeth.) They are not significant and they'll disappear within ten to fourteen days.

Some babies are born with teeth in their mouth. The teeth may be apparent immediately, or may appear one or two days after birth. Usually these are not extra teeth but are the primary teeth, which are forming very close to the mucosa. If the baby is healthy and the teeth do not interfere with nursing or cause lesions on the tongue, they should be left in place. There is no reason to feel that the child will aspirate the tooth if he is healthy and has all his protective mechanisms.

Later, small cysts may develop on the gum pads. These are the sacs that surround a developing tooth. They are called "eruption cysts," and tend to disappear after a few days. Don't let anyone cut or puncture them. They have poor circulation and can easily become infected.

BEFORE THE FIRST TOOTH

Immediately after the baby's birth, parents can start to do something about their child's teeth. What they do during the first year will set the stage for what happens to his teeth for the rest of his life. It's not too early to think about the permanent teeth, which start to form right after birth. These permanent teeth are developing in the baby's jaw while you are waiting for his first primary tooth to erupt, or appear.

Statistics indicate that if your child is going to get a cavity in his primary teeth, it will be on the biting surface of the first primary molar or on the side of that primary tooth. These are the very areas that are developing during the first three years of life. If he's going to get a cavity in his permanent teeth, the story is exactly the same — the biting surface and side are the most vulnerable, and they, too, are developing from birth on. Try to think of these areas as especially caries-sensitive. The best method of protecting them is to get fluoride into them.

Fluoride for Infants

If babies knew what was good for them, they'd howl for fluoride. "No problem," say the parents, reassuringly. "Our community's water supply is fluoridated." Fine, but if you are breast-feeding your child and he is not getting a supplemental bottle, he is probably not getting any fluoride. Mother's milk contains almost no fluoride, even if the mother is drinking water that contains fluoride. Just as long as the child starts getting water mixed in his food when he is around six months, there is no problem. Studies today indicate that there is no reason to supplement a child's fluoride intake if he lives in an area that has fluoridated water even though he is being breast-fed. Fluoride supplements given to an infant living in such an area can cause fluorosis. This is a condition in which white spots develop on the front surface of the permanent teeth. The spots are caused by too much fluoride ingested too early.

It had previously been assumed that infants living in communities with nonfluoridated drinking water would be likely to receive only a small amount of fluoride each day. However, a lot of recent research suggests that even in these areas infants are receiving more dietary fluoride than was previously thought. Commercially prepared concentrated liquid formulas often contain quantities of fluoride. The amount varies among products, even those produced by the same manufacturer, since the products may be made in plants in different cities.

Whether an appropriate single daily dose of fluoride beginning at birth confers significantly greater protection against dental caries than does an appropriate single daily dose of fluoride beginning when the baby is six months old is currently unknown. In view of this uncertainty it is extremely difficult to ascertain what is an appropriate daily dose of fluoride for infants less than six months of age. It seems to me desirable to sometimes delay fluoride supplementation until the baby is six months old.

SINGLE DAILY DOSE OF FLUORIDE

Because of the many children who do not have access to fluoridated drinking water, the effectiveness of single daily doses of fluoride is a matter of considerable interest. Without question, a single daily dose of fluoride in either drop or tablet form will substantially reduce the caries-attack rate. Combined fluoride-vitamin preparations are readily acceptable forms for providing the proper dosage. If your baby is receiving vitamins, use one of the vitamin preparations that contain fluoride. They seem to provide an effective means of getting fluoride to the teeth. Purists in fluoride therapy claim that if the fluoride is taken in the form of a large tablet or lozenge, it will impart additional benefits by a topical effect on the teeth.

The purpose of single-dose fluoride, of course, is to achieve maximal protection against dental caries with minimal risk of fluorosis of the enamel. Every community's water supply differs in the amount of naturally occurring flouride. I believe that during the next few years modifications in dosages for infants will be made, so I suggest that you find a knowledgeable local physician or dentist and have him help you determine how much fluoride your child should get.

Try to Keep Your Baby Well

Of course, you'd do this anyway, but there is an important connection between general health and teeth. An infectious illness or a high fever affects the adjustment of calcium and phosphorous salts in the baby's bloodstream. This means that the primary and permanent teeth developing at this time will mineralize imperfectly. Poor enamel and dentine crystals form, causing the teeth to be more susceptible to cavities.

If you've been thinking that certain childhood diseases are inevitable and that it's best to go ahead and "get them over with," then it's time to change your mind. *Prevent childhood diseases* until your child is three and a half or four. Give those teeth a chance to form.

If your baby is ill during the first year, there are two things to remember:

- Try to avoid giving your baby tetracycline. Today there are good alternative antibiotics. Tetracycline, especially during the first year of life, will stain primary and permanent teeth.
- Keep a record of childhood illnesses. If your baby is ill during his first year, before his first tooth erupts into the mouth, special care will have to be taken to keep his mouth clean. The teeth may come into the mouth looking fine to the mother and father — and even to the dentist. But because of imperfect mineralization, these teeth may have a congenital susceptibility to caries. When your child goes to the dentist for the first time, make a point of giving him or her information about childhood illnesses, so that it becomes part of your child's record.

PACIFIERS

Pacifiers come in all shapes and sizes. The thumb and the fingers are the ones that nature provides; the rubber and plastic models from the drugstore are provided by Mom and Dad.

Right from birth — and even before — most babies have an urge to suck on anything that is placed in or near the mouth. This is an inborn, natural reflex and should not be discouraged. Many babies get enough sucking by nursing or using a bottle with a proper nipple (that is, a non-free-flowing type). Other babies seem to need more of this activity.

Research, to date, indicates that children should be encouraged to work the muscles in their tongue and cheeks, and to exercise the swallowing reflex as much and as soon as possible, in order to get their muscles into proper balance and thus develop a musculature that will lead the teeth into the mouth in a straight, even position. Further, the child who sucks vigorously and is given an opportunity to practice his chewing is preparing a good environment for his primary teeth to erupt into. Teeth don't know where they're going — there's no game plan. Have you seen, in the bottom front teeth of an older child, the permanent tooth that comes in behind the front primary central? The tongue begins to push that tooth forward, the lips hold it back, and the dynamics of the mouth encourage it to go where it's needed.

Children should be encouraged to chew and bite as soon as possible — even before the first tooth comes into the mouth. For many children, teething rings and toys and natural foods can serve this purpose. If your child uses a pacifier, don't worry. If he doesn't lose it or forget it before his permanent incisors erupt, *then* begin to worry (see pages 43–44). The only advantage of an artificial over a natural pacifier (thumb, fingers) is that it is likely to be lost, and at some future date the habit will more easily be given up. How forceful the parents can be at that time without disturbing their relationship with the child and with each other is an important consideration. Try to evaluate the problem on a rational basis.

The effect that the pacifier habit will have on teeth is usually proportional to the amount of time the child has worked at the habit. Accordingly, three hours a day is better than five hours, two years is better than three years, and this, in turn, is better than allowing the child to continue the habit into his fourth or fifth year. If a child can be encouraged to work at it less and less each day, he'll have fewer problems later. Since children go to sleep before their mothers and fathers, the parents can remove the pacifier or thumb from the sleeping child's mouth every time one of them passes his bed.

My Best Suggestions for Breaking Bad Habits

Step 1: Understand, first, that a habit is an unconscious muscular pattern. It must be brought to conscious attention before it can be dealt with. If your child sucks his thumb, tell him so: "Johnny, you're sucking your thumb." Don't be negative — he has no control over the habit because he doesn't know he's sucking. It may take three or four months before Johnny *knows* that he's putting his thumb in his mouth.

Step 2: After he understands that he has a habit, and agrees that it would be better not to stick his thumb in his mouth, you may suggest aids that will remind him — anything from an appliance made by a dentist to a piece of tape placed on the thumb as a reminder, or a sock on the hand when he goes to sleep. To use any of these aids before the child is aware of the habit and agrees that he really wants to drop it is going to do more harm than good.

Habits such as tongue-thrusting and lip-biting take a long time to break — perhaps as long as two or three years. But the effort is well worth it. It takes no longer than the orthodontics that may be ahead if the habit is not left behind by the maturing child.

Try to adopt a relaxed but firm attitude about it. Understand that you're dealing with a habit: the longer it is practiced, the more difficult it will be to stop. Think of a habit as a series of unconscious muscular movements that are repeated over and over. To stop a habit, you must first bring it to a conscious level. This is best done by gently, yet persistently, reminding a child that she is engaging in the habit each time she does so. Again, be gentle. Don't put a value on it; don't imply that "bad children suck their thumbs, good children do not." No rewards. Just stay loose, and remember that eventually most children get the idea. In fact, most children give up this habit by age three or four without any parental guidance at all.

Of all malocclusions — faulty closures of the teeth — that occur, those caused solely by thumb-sucking or pacifiers are the easiest to correct. But if you'd rather avoid them now than correct them later, here are the points to remember:

- The longer a child continues a habit, the greater the chance for malocclusion to develop.
- All children need to suck and bite. But when such activity is carried on for prolonged periods of time, it becomes a pernicious habit. The earlier it is stopped (preferably by the time the child is two and a half years old), the less damage it will do. Damage to the dentition is a function of time. The longer the child retains the habit, the more damage he does.
- If the habit is still present after the permanent teeth start to erupt, you've got a serious problem.

Often a dentist examining a child for the first time will count the child's fingers before looking at his teeth. This allows the dentist to make body contact gradually, and in a nonthreatening area of the body. It gets the child's attention. And it gives the dentist information. When the dentist sees a clean thumb or finger, he knows the child has a built-in pacifier.

A child with a strong, persistent urge to suck will sometimes substitute other activities as he grows older. See the section on bad habits, pages 38–44, for a fuller discussion.

NURSING

One of the purposes of the baby's nursing (besides the obvious one of obtaining nourishment) is educating the muscles of the lips, cheeks, tongue, and jaw to more and more mature ways of handling fuel for the body. These muscles, along with taste buds, heat-sensitive nerve endings, and salivary glands (and later the teeth), make up the mouth's apparatus for evaluating, manipulating, masticating, and swallowing food.

Nursing affects the development of muscular patterns. If an unnatural pattern is formed, the erupting teeth will not be directed into the proper position, and the child may develop a malocclusion.

Breast or Bottle?

The breast-fed child must work the tongue and the muscles around the mouth vigorously, in a pattern perfected throughout the evolutionary process. It's quite a skilled activity. In addition, when the child is nursing from the breast, he is generally held upright — the natural position, with gravity working correctly on the muscles. A mother may decide to nurse her child until all the anterior primary teeth are in, at about the age of two. Once the primary teeth are in, the tongue adapts to the shape of the teeth, the swallowing pattern changes, and the child is ready to move on to new foods.

When the baby is nursing from a breast substitute — a bottle, that is — the action is entirely different. Milk is not supplied on demand but often flows from the bottle in a continuous stream. The muscles of the mouth don't work as hard, and if the baby nurses while lying on his back, he must keep his tongue in an unnatural forward position to keep himself from drowning!

Nursing Checklist

1. If your baby uses a bottle, encourage him to stay in an upright position while nursing.
2. Use a bottle with a nipple that has a small hole. Check to see that the baby is required to work to get milk from the bottle. There are several kinds of nipples on the market. Find a type that is non-free-flowing and makes the child move his cheeks, tongue, and jaws. Most orthodontic problems in young children are caused by an imbalance in musculature.
3. Introduce the child to drinking from a cup as soon as possible.
4. Let the baby feed from the bottle at intervals, as though it were a breast.
5. Day or night, *never use a nursing bottle as a pacifier.* Milk or juice that constantly bathes the teeth will cause severe cavities.
6. Clean the mouth and teeth at least once a day.

If you breast-feed for a while and then wean the baby to a bottle and not to a cup, observe the foregoing rules. Bad habits start as early as birth and can be initiated any time thereafter.

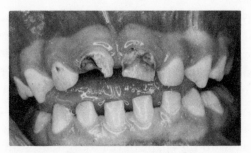

Cindy — three years old

Cindy is still using a bottle. She walks around with it during the day. Her mother says Cindy likes chocolate milk best. Had the mother given her water instead, there would be no damage to Cindy's teeth.

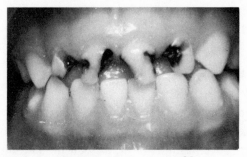

Tommy — two years old

Tommy was given a bottle of apple juice every night when he went to bed.

THE DANGER OF USING A NURSING BOTTLE AS A PACIFIER

The front teeth of two preschool children show the destruction that can occur to the upper front teeth when a child is allowed to sleep with a bottle or to walk around during the day with the bottle in his or her mouth.

Nursing-Bottle Mouth

What's the worst thing you can do to a brand-new baby?

1. Forget his vitamins.
2. Drop him on his head.
3. Stick him in his crib with a bottle at nap time or let him walk around during the day with a bottle in his mouth.

A dentist would choose Number 3. Tooth decay is practically epidemic among children who have been allowed to use a bottle as a pacifier. (The pictures opposite illustrate the danger.)

In these children, widespread decay is found in all the upper teeth and sometimes in lower back teeth, but almost never in the lower front teeth. That's because when the child is nursing, the tongue covers and protects the lower teeth while the nipple is pressed between the top surface of the tongue and the upper jaw.

If a child is allowed to have a bottle and go to sleep with it, as he sleeps milk or juice in the mouth and on the teeth turns to acid and causes the teeth to start to break down very rapidly. Although cavities may not appear until the fourth or fifth year of life, they can be caused by the baby's having slept with a nursing bottle for long periods of time.

If your baby is still using a nursing bottle when his teeth begin to appear, let him use it for short periods of time, awake and sitting up. If he is using a bottle for a pacifier, put water in the bottle. Not only is water harmless to teeth, but if the baby has not been drinking local fluoridated water because he had something else in his bottle, now is the chance to get fluoridated water into his diet.

Unprepared as you may be for it, decay can actually start in primary teeth when the child is between eight and twenty-four months. The American Society of Dentistry for Children tells us that 50 percent of all two-year-olds have at least one cavity. The possibility of decay occurring at such an early age is increased by the following practices:

- The child is permitted to go to sleep with a bottle containing milk, juice, or a sweetened drink.
- The child is permitted to have a bottle containing juice or sweet-

ened milk throughout the day, long after he has learned to drink
from a cup.

- Parents give the baby a pacifier dipped in honey, jelly, or sugar.
  If such an outrageous impulse occurs to you, block it.
- The child is two years of age and no one has ever cleaned his
  teeth.

If a child two or younger comes into my office with cavities, I
know before he even sits in my chair that one of the above practices
is the cause.

We can see from statistics what effect the bottle habit can have on
the incidence of decay in primary teeth. The average three- to four-
year-old has one to two and a half decayed-filled teeth. A child whose
dental deterioration traces back to many hours spent with juice or
formula bathing his teeth can expect to have more than ten decayed-
filled teeth in his primary set. When your child grows beyond the
bottle-feeding age, get rid of the bottle.

EARLY CLEANING ROUTINE

If we could get rid of plaque, most of our problems would be over.
But as long as we harbor bacteria in our mouths (and we do), and
as long as we continue to put food into our mouths (and we will),
we're going to have plaque. It is an almost invisible film, containing
a sticky substance, that coats the teeth and sets the stage for dental
decay and gum disease. The oral bacteria that live in plaque, reacting
with various food residues, excrete an acid that, held to the tooth in
the sticky film, goes to work to break down the tooth structure.
Plaque must be carefully removed every day from the mouth of
anyone who intends to have healthy teeth and gums.

It is possible that you won't take your child to the dentist for his
first visit before he is three or four years old. That's one reason I've
written this book: I want to get information into your hands immediately.

Cleaning should begin when your child has a tooth in his mouth.
The gum pads in your child's mouth are covered with the same
tissue that covers newly erupted teeth. The colonies of bacteria that

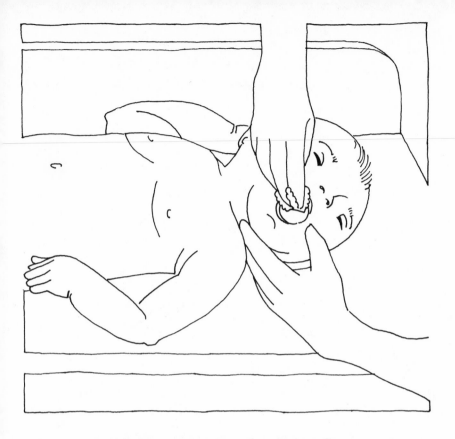

HOW TO CLEAN AN INFANT'S TEETH. *See page 21.*

form on the gum pads are the same as those that form on the erupting teeth. By keeping the gum pads clean, you can remove food residues. You can also reduce the oral bacteria and cut down on the acid produced.

With less acid in her mouth, the baby will have an easier time teething; with a lower bacteria count, she may even have fewer colds during her first year. And her first teeth will arrive in a clean, plaque-free environment.

A piece of gauze (2″ × 2″) held between the thumb and forefinger and wiped vigorously over the ridge of the top and bottom jaws is an effective cleaner and plaque remover. The easiest position for you to be in when carrying out this procedure is to keep the baby's head in your lap, feet pointing away. The cleaning should be done twice a day — after breakfast and after the last meal in the evening. It should take about two minutes to do.

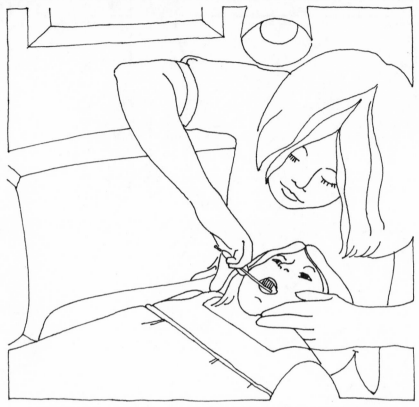

HOW TO CLEAN A CHILD'S TEETH. *See opposite page.*

The use of a dentifrice is optional. It will bring some fluoride in contact with the tooth. The main purpose here is to get the film (plaque) off the teeth, if a dentifrice gets in your way, don't use it.

Use just enough pressure to remove the film that is covering the child's teeth. It should be about as much pressure as you would need to squeeze a fresh marshmallow between your fingers. Think of the action of your fingers as being the same as squeezing the marshmallow. There is some evidence that this kind of cleaning routine can help reduce teething pain.

This simple step is one of the foundations of early prevention. It is the parents' responsibility, for the child can no more do it than he can clean his ears or trim his nails. And yet, simple as it is, it involves a complex behavioral change on the part of parents, because it means adding a habit to your life that was not part of your own growing up and that is probably not observed by your peers.

The Best Way to Examine and Clean Your Child's Teeth

If you are going to become familiar with your child's teeth and keep them clean, as suggested in this book, there is a good position for you to assume when doing so. Seat yourself on the floor, or on a couch or bed, with the child lying down in front of you, her head on your lap, her feet facing away, the crown of her head facing toward your navel. This is the only way you can see clearly her back teeth, both top and bottom. If you try to look in while facing the child directly, her lips and tongue get in the way and you can't see — or brush — effectively.

Another method of examining a child's mouth is to take a piece of gauze, like the piece you used to wipe the baby's teeth, and put it on the tip of the child's tongue, holding it between your fingers and moving it to the right and left, so that you can get a look. Still another way is to use a small pocket flashlight while you hold and move the tongue with a spoon. You'll be surprised at how much you can see.

It's a simple matter, and it can be fun, to check the number of teeth, their color, see if surfaces are clean, and help your child with brushing. I'm always amazed at the number of parents bringing their children to my office who have never themselves looked at their children's teeth. What's the hangup?

Many parents are afraid to look into a child's mouth; they regard the mouth as part of the inside of the body and, therefore, somehow inaccessible. They have no cultural excuse for such a procedure (their friends don't do it, their parents didn't do it). And they fear they are going to introduce some infection. (Did you ever try to make a list of the things that go in and out of a baby's mouth every day? A clean piece of gauze on his mother's finger is nothing!)

Some parents who do this for the first time notice a tiny bit of bleeding of the child's gums. This doesn't mean they're pushing too hard; it means the gum tissue was already irritated. Keep at it for a few days — the condition will clear up.

So you can see that, because of these objections and feelings, it's going to take some effort on your part to get as interested in cleaning the mouth as you are in cleaning and caring for other parts of the child's body. Although the baby may object initially, mothers who have adopted the routine find that the child begins to enjoy it and that it can be done rapidly and effectively.

CHEWING

What did babies eat before there were formulas and pabulum and baby foods?

For thousands of years, children began to eat available, natural foods about the time they gave up nursing. Hard to believe, isn't it?

Children can be encouraged to get into the habit of chewing before any teeth erupt into their mouths. The gum pads provide children with strong biting surfaces. They serve the same purpose as the toothless ridges in a sixty-year-old who goes on enjoying a varied diet. *Children can chew food without teeth.* Teeth are not that important for chewing. Healthy children have amazing reflexes that will prevent them from swallowing food they cannot handle. As soon as a child is able to grasp food, he should be encouraged to chew it. The tougher the food, the harder its consistency, the better it will be for the child. Lazy chewing habits cause caries and — this may surprise you — malocclusion. Possibly one of the greatest causes of orthodontic problems is that children today are kept on soft foods for such long periods of time, just when their muscles and neuromuscular pathways are developing.

Just as many child psychologists believe that personality traits are developed when children are very young, many pediatric dentists think that preferences for soft foods (which will not naturally clean the teeth and will cause more cavities) and lazy chewing habits (which will lead to crooked teeth) are developed with the solicitous help of attentive parents, who mistakenly weed out hard foods and feed their children soft foods — sometimes even after the children are twelve months old.

If you are willing to try, you will find that children as young as seven or eight months can and will chew when given the chance. Try

Some Hints for Dealing with Swallowed Objects:

1. Is the child choking or having difficulty breathing? If not, he's probably swallowed the object and it's in his stomach. If it's the size of a nickel or smaller, it's potentially no more serious than a swallowed cherry pit.
2. If the child is having difficulty breathing, turn him upside down and with your finger try to dislodge the object caught in his throat.
3. If you can't dislodge the object that way, and if the child is small enough, pick him up by the heels and shake him vigorously.
4. If the child is too big to pick up and shake, take a position behind him with your arms around his lower chest. Join your hands and jerk hard. The air below will be forced against the diaphragm, which will react by snapping upward and ejecting the object.

If you are unable to deal with it yourself, remember that most objects don't fit the throat perfectly — they don't completely cut off air. You usually have time to get to the emergency room of your local hospital or to summon emergency treatment.

introducing to the baby's diet such challenging foods as carrots and celery strips, chewy toast, and crisp apple and pear slices.

MOUTH INFECTIONS

As you become more familiar with the geography of your baby's mouth, you'll be quicker to notice anything unusual going on there. In general, the mouth has great resistance to infection. If the baby does get an infection of the mouth, it will usually be either cold sores or thrush. Both infections are often associated with high fever.

Thrush (moniliasis) is recognized by white patches on the tongue and lips; it should be treated with antibiotics.

Cold sores (herpes, stomatitis) generally develop around the lips and inside the mouth, and often look like little bubbles at first. The lesions usually last eight to ten days, and there is no medicine that will help shorten the period of time, so a philosophical attitude is recommended. Don't give the child spicy foods and acidic foods, such as orange juice — and *no mouthwashes.* You can provide a little short-term relief if there are small, isolated lesions on cheeks and lips: dry them and place small dabs of Vaseline on them.

TONGUE-TIE

At birth, and for a few days after, there is in the mouth a little membrane that "ties" the tongue to the mandibular ridge. This membrane places the tongue in the proper position for the child to nurse; during nursing the nipple is compressed between the upper gum pad and the top of the tongue. The membrane usually disappears in a few days, and the child is able to stretch the tongue forward.

In some instances, the membrane turns into heavy tissue and the tip of the tongue is locked into position and cannot be extended. This condition has been known to cause problems with the position of the erupting teeth.

When the child is about four months of age, she should be checked by her parents, who can tell if she is able stick the tip of her tongue over her front teeth, in the direction of her nose. How? Try making faces, encouraging the child to imitate you.

THE SPECIAL CHILD

Some children come into the world with a handicap or disability that is the result of illness or a congenital deformity. A child who is dentally handicapped is a child who has massive caries, a cleft palate, or a trauma — broken and injured teeth. A child who is handicapped for dentistry has a mental or physical problem that makes him unable to cope with ordinary dental procedures.

Just as parents and child adapt to the special demands of such a child's condition, they must set themselves the task of giving special care to the child's teeth. If dental problems are allowed to develop, they will be harder to treat because of the child's other problem.

Children with heart disease, cerebral palsy, mental retardation, and other conditions deserve an extra dose of care. A hemophiliac, for example, who can't take an injection should not have to spend ten weeks of his life in hospitals before he is eight years old for dental care alone — which he can expect to do if his teeth haven't received careful attention.

When a child is ill, parents tend to become oversolicitous. They will often feed the child constantly, let him use a bottle as a pacifier, and keep him on soft foods for a long period of time — all of which will complicate the dental situation.

Think about it. If you've got one serious problem already, you don't need another.

The handicapped child may, when he's older, need to go more often to the dentist for observation and evaluation. This will bring two benefits:

- The child learns, through familiarity, to be less anxious and more cooperative at the dentist's office.
- Frequent checkups reduce the need for extensive treatment, which might involve admitting the child to the hospital for dental treatment under general anesthesia, a costly procedure and a potentially dangerous one. A two- or three-year-old is a poor anesthesia risk compared to a ten-year old. If the choice is made to use anesthesia — and I do sometimes make that choice — you'll want the best possible anesthesiologist because the dentistry is the easy part. It's putting a baby to sleep that's tough.

Review the caries checklist on page 114. Remember, since most dental disease *is* preventable, handicapped children, especially, should not be its victims.

The baby is now five or six months old. He has a clean, plaque-free mouth; he is getting fluorides in the water he drinks or is about to begin a fluoride supplement; he chews vigorously and with evident pleasure when he's handed a piece of crisp celery or chewy toast; and he's beginning to feel little tingly sensations in the ridge of gum in the front of his mouth. Could it be that he is about to produce a surprise for Mom and Dad and Grandma and Grandpa and all the rest?

TWO

From First Tooth to Adult Tooth

One day your baby looks up at you and smiles, and there, gleaming like perfect pearls, are a couple of brand-new teeth. The first teeth generally come into the mouth when the child is between six and fourteen months old. They may be the two center front teeth on the bottom or the two center front on the top — the incisors. They are small, even, and very white (in fact, so white that when the big, strong, yellowish permanent teeth begin to come in, it will take you a while to get used to the contrast). When all four front incisors are in, the lateral incisors — the very small teeth on either side of the front center teeth — will make their appearance, probably two at a time.

Some children get their teeth early; some children get their teeth late. There's really no medical importance attached to the timing. Every baby has his own schedule, and it may safely vary from the chart on page 30. The chart is just to give you an idea of the standard progression, using average ages of eruption. Your child's age may deviate as much as ten to twelve months and still be within the normal range.

There is really no significance to either early or late eruption, except that those children whose teeth erupt later tend to have a higher resistance to dental caries than those whose teeth erupt earlier. In part this is because teeth that stay under gums for a longer time in areas where there is fluoride in the water supply will pick up more fluoride from body tissues before they come out to face the world.

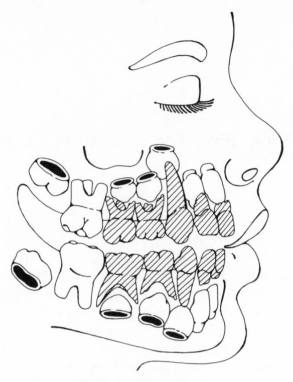

HOW TEETH GROW

This child has his primary teeth and his first permanent molars. The other permanent teeth have not yet erupted.

In general, girls' teeth tend to erupt slightly before boys' teeth do. That's no advantage; we shall see later that girls show somewhat more susceptibility than boys to early dental caries, probably because their teeth have been out longer, exposed to things that can cause decay.

By the time some children are fourteen months old, they have four teeth in their mouth, others of the same age (like my two sons) are just beginning to show their first tooth. Keep an eye on what's going on in there: the progression of teething and the number of teeth in your baby's mouth shouldn't be a mystery.

Before your baby is three, certain things may come to your attention that you'll want to consult a dentist about. Your baby may develop too few teeth. This is sometimes an inherited condition. An x-ray will reveal if the teeth really are missing or are just late in coming through. Your baby may have too many teeth. If there has been some malformation of the enamel and the teeth look chalky and white with brownish areas, or are soft with yellow spots, special care will have to be taken to reinforce and save these teeth. Most babies of eighteen months have approximately twelve teeth. By the time the baby is three years old, he should have twenty teeth in his mouth: ten in the bottom jaw and ten in the upper jaw. Twenty — count 'em — twenty. Missing and extra teeth are not uncommon and can very often lead to malocclusions if they are not detected early. Check with your dentist. Teeth can erupt malformed or out of alignment, or not appear at all. Or an early cavity may develop.

The illustration on page 28 shows the mouth at three years with all twenty teeth accounted for. There should be four teeth in between each of the pointed canine teeth and then the first and second molars on each side. If there are fewer — or more — after the third birthday, there is reason for concern.

TEETHING

Although there is wide variation in individual teething patterns, statistics indicate a general progression. The first teeth to come into the mouth are usually the lower central incisors, followed by the top central incisors. The chart opposite shows the pattern that occurs most frequently. Your baby might vary by several months and there would still be no reason to worry.

Once the central incisors are in, your child will be teething off and on for the next two years. When he's around nine months old, the lateral incisors (the teeth next to the central incisors) arrive. When he's between twelve and fourteen months, the first molars erupt, leaving a gap that the canines will fill at about eighteen months. By the time he's two, the second molars have come in. Then there will be a long waiting period until he is five or six, when those very important teeth, the six-year molars, arrive.

Erik Erikson has made a guess that the legend of the Garden of Eden, which is told in one version or another by all peoples of the world, goes back to the common preverbal experience when a fussy, cranky, teething baby bites down on his mother's breast, precipitat-

Life Cycle of the Primary Teeth

Tooth	When It Arrives (Month)*	When It Leaves (Year)
The upper teeth		
Central incisor	7.5	7
Lateral incisor	9	8
Cuspid	18	11
First molar	14	9
Second molar	24	11
The lower teeth		
Central incisor	6	6
Lateral incisor	7	7
Cuspid	16	10
First molar	12	9
Second molar	20	10

*Plus or minus six months should be considered to be within the normal limit.

ing her decision that it's time to wean the baby and resulting in the child's sense of loss of a paradise.

Teething is only one of the stresses a baby is going through at the active, adventurous age of six months to one year. If a six-month-old has two temper tantrums, throws up on Grandpa's lap, and screams his head off for no apparent reason, his parents might be tempted to shrug their shoulders and explain, "He must be teething." It seems as if every time a child whines, drools, cries, or puts things into his mouth, somebody is bound to blame it on teething. And since teeth are erupting off and on from six months to three years, there would hardly be a time when it couldn't be blamed.

If your child is giving some of these signals, take a look in her mouth. The first teeth to arrive will be front and center (the four central incisors erupt around the sixth to the tenth month). If the gums here look irritated, red, and puffy, and if you can feel or even see the tip of a tooth coming through, then your baby is teething. If other symptoms show up (fever, nausea, congestion), don't assume that teething is the cause — *real* sickness is not caused by teething. Check with your pediatrician for other possibilities.

If you don't see any teeth but would like to know where they are, press your thumb firmly on the gum tissue and take it away, quickly; you'll see the shape of the tooth underneath for just a second.

There is a great deal of controversy about whether there is any pain associated with teething. There probably is none. Teeth don't really "cut" through the gums. The process is one of gradual movement. Teething is a perfectly natural process, running on an individual timetable. In my seventeen years of experience as a children's dentist, I have never found it necessary to cut a child's gums to help the primary teeth come through.

If there is some discomfort in teething, different measures seem to relieve it in different babies; you'll find them through experience and observation. I once handed a teething baby a cold, cooked, shelled shrimp, and it worked; but I don't prescribe it, since I don't know whether it was the texture, the temperature, or the novelty of the remedy that worked.

The best thing to do for a teething baby is to clean her mouth with a damp gauze pad three or four times a day and give her something to bite on — a teething ring, toast, a chicken drumstick bone stripped of meat.

If your child seems to lose her appetite for a while, don't worry. Don't use coercion to get her to eat. You wouldn't force a pet dog or cat — or an adult, for that matter — to eat if he or she was obviously resisting the idea, would you? Let the child decide.

Drooling

It is not unusual for healthy children to drool. When a child is very young, he does not have the muscular control to keep saliva in his mouth. Many things stimulate excessive saliva production: foods, smells, strange tastes, or the irritation that develops around a newly erupted tooth that hasn't been properly cleaned.

THOSE IMPORTANT PRIMARY TEETH

It wouldn't bother me as a dentist not to meet a child before he was three if I thought that child's parents were keeping his gum pads clean and continuing the daily cleaning habit as the new primary teeth came into the mouth, taking gauze or cloth and wiping the new teeth, as well as the gum pads, after meals to clear away food and keep plaque from forming. But many people still feel that the primary teeth are not important because they are going to fall out anyway. Let's examine that idea a little more carefully.

The twenty primary teeth are designed to function during the childhood years — some of them until the child is ten or twelve — and they have several important jobs to do.

1. Primary teeth are responsible for maintaining proper spaces for the child's permanent teeth to come into; they serve to guide permanent teeth into position.
2. They help in the development of the face and jaws, influencing the growth, height, and shape of the face. How many of us have seen an adult whose face seemed to collapse when he took out his set of dentures? Teeth contribute to one's appearance and sense of self-worth.
3. These primary teeth certainly help in the first step of digesting food — and now the baby is changing his diet to more solid fare, foods that need biting and chewing and grinding.
4. Healthy, decay-free primary teeth create an environment of healthy flora for the permanent teeth.

Do you begin to see how important the first teeth are? Instead of thinking of "primary" in its narrow meaning of "first," think of the word as describing a fundamental, basic, important part of an organized whole. *Primary* teeth are *foundation* teeth. Early neglect or early loss can result in several problems, and you may as well think about them while you still have a chance to prevent them.

There was a time when dentists thought that all prematurely lost primary teeth had to be replaced, but it's not so. For example, in the upper anterior region spaces don't close up. In fact, as a child gets older and his jaw gets bigger, spaces open up with or without teeth to hold them.

But in some areas of the mouth, particularly the posterior part, the premature loss of a primary tooth may mean trouble. The adjacent teeth tend to drift into this space; the leaning, crooked teeth will collect more food and be more susceptible to decay. And the drifted tooth may block a permanent tooth that is waiting to move into that space, or may cause it to erupt at an angle as it tries to find a place for itself. Teeth don't know where they are going; if they did, we wouldn't have coined the word "malocclusion," and orthodontists would have to find some other specialty to practice.

- Injuries to the front primary teeth can cause infections and disturbances in the development of the permanent front teeth.
- Of course primary teeth fall out. In fact, the front teeth are kept only five or six years. But some of the posterior primary teeth will be in the mouth for a long time, sometimes until the child is eleven or twelve years of age. If these teeth are carrying dental disease — caries — they will pass it right along to the new permanent teeth. If a sound six-year molar, which is a permanent tooth, erupts into a mouth that is already harboring caries, it will not take long for the new tooth to be affected, for decay travels fast.
- If a primary tooth becomes infected and abscessed at the root, the infection may damage the underlying permanent tooth.
- If a primary tooth is removed, instead of being filled and saved, expensive braces or space maintainers may be needed to save the space for the unerupted permanent tooth. Whether a space maintainer is needed is generally a dentist's decision.
- The six-year molar — the first permanent tooth to appear in the mouth — is going to be the key to the placement of the permanent teeth. It is important, therefore, for the first and second primary molars to be healthy teeth, present and in their normal position, so that this all-important six-year molar can come into its correct position in the dental arch.

A Look at Primary Teeth

The hard outer coat of the baby's tooth is the enamel, and the part you see is called the crown. The inner, supportive structure, which you cannot see, is the dentin. All of that part of the tooth was formed in the uterus and was in the jaw when the baby was born. However, the root, which anchors the tooth and holds it in position, wasn't developed enough to do that job until about the sixth or eighth month after birth. This is all part of nature's timetable.

Color: The color of the first tooth that comes into the mouth is an indication of what the color of all the other teeth is going to be. If the mother was not ill during pregnancy, there is no reason for it not to be a milky-white color. If it is some other color, it may indicate a malformation of the enamel, and a dentist should be consulted.

In general, a stained primary tooth probably has the stain not in the tooth but on the outside of the tooth. A stain of this kind can be removed very easily with a piece of gauze and a little dentifrice.

Mamelons — "Little Bumps": The first tooth will have small bumps on the biting surface. These are called "mamelons." They do not constitute a cutting edge to help the tooth get through the gum, as some people believe. Rather, they are simply the areas where the tooth buds start to develop. A lower incisor will have three or four mamelons on it. In general, these mamelons are worn away as the teeth come into contact with the teeth in the opposing jaw. Mamelons that have *not* worn away after a few years are an indication that the teeth are not being used properly. Malocclusion is probably starting to develop. So watch and see if the mamelons start to disappear by the second or third birthday.

Frenum: That little flap of tissue that attaches the center of each lip to the jaw is called the "frenum." In some children the flap seems to sit between the permanent incisors, and there may be some space between these two front teeth. A dentist may suggest excising the frenum so that this space can close. In my experience, the need for such surgery is very infrequent. This tissue is not necessarily what's keeping the teeth apart.

On rare occasions the frenum is a heavy, tough band — it looks like a rubber band, doubled over — connected on the tongue side. Then it does have to be removed surgically, but it's a simple procedure, with no deleterious effects. In the lower jaw, the frenum may be attached right at the neck of the lower incisors. In that position it pulls at the tissue, and is a sufficiently severe problem to require surgical repair. If this is the case, have the surgery done when the child is around nine or ten. Once the child is over fourteen or fifteen, the periodontal problem is irreversible. A specialist in gum surgery — a periodontist — usually handles a frenectomy.

Spaces: Does your baby have spaces between his new teeth? It's actually an advantage, for primary teeth with natural separation are less likely to harbor food particles and are consequently less susceptible to decay. Nature meant teeth to be self-cleaning: straight, spaced, washed by saliva, and scoured by the coarse, unrefined foods people ate for centuries. Even if your child's teeth don't seem well spaced when they first come in, you will notice that when he's about five years old the upper primary teeth begin to spread apart a little. The growing jaw is providing room for the larger permanent teeth, which will eventually take the place of the primary teeth.

CLEANING THE FIRST TEETH

A child can't clean his own mouth efficiently — any more than he can pick up a pen and write script or cut his food neatly by manipulating his knife and fork. The neural patterns and the muscular coordination that he needs for maintaining good hygiene do not develop until he is eight or nine years old. So the skills it takes to manipulate the toothbrush and dental floss are just not there; he can't clean his own teeth thoroughly. Therefore, you're responsible for keeping your child's mouth clean, and you're stuck with the task for a long time. Meanwhile, you're establishing a behavior pattern in both the child and yourself.

Think your own attitude through clearly: this is not something you are doing *to* your child but something you are doing *for* your child. The child knows the difference. You are not a tyrant, pinning your child to the wall forcibly to brush his teeth; you are a parent who cares about his child's body, showing him in visible and physical terms that you do, and indicating to him that it is important that he, too, learn to value and care for his physical well-being.

The cleaning ritual should take place after the first meal in the morning and after the last meal at night.

Many children are still nursing from a bottle when their teeth begin to come into their mouth. I have already alerted you to the dangers of letting your child nurse for long periods of time or allowing him to take a bottle of juice or milk into his bed at night. There is really no need to feed children constantly. Isn't your child getting an adequate diet at mealtime?

Once the teeth start to erupt into the mouth, they should be cleaned exactly as you've been cleaning the gum pads. Use the position described on page 19. The cleaning should entail the wiping of both surfaces — front and back — of the teeth with a gauze pad held between the fingers. Continue to clean the gum pads, too. As other teeth erupt into the mouth, clean gum pads will keep the area clean and free of food particles, and will cut down on the number of bacteria in the mouth. If the teeth start to stain, a little bit of a fluoride dentifrice approved by the American Dental Association's Council on Dental Therapeutics can be used on the gauze pads.

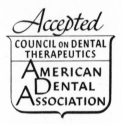

At some point — after the incisors are in — you'll want to graduate to a small toothbrush with a straight, small head and even, soft bristles. You will still have to do most of the brushing for some time.

As the child approaches his second birthday, he can be introduced to using a toothbrush himself. However, this is just to get him into the habit of holding his toothbrush and brushing — a good habit to develop. Good dental habits established with the primary teeth will usually be carried over into the care of the permanent teeth. But for now, it is still neither his job nor his responsibility to keep his mouth clean. Few children before the age of seven can do an adequate job of cleaning their mouths.

My experience has always been that the parent wants the child to be independent and take care of his own teeth. Instinctively — more important, culturally — parents don't want to feel responsible for cleaning their children's teeth. When I counsel parents I suggest to them, "Look at it this way — you're helping your child to reach a point where he can manage by himself."

You may want to use a little dentifrice on the gauze pad or on a soft brush after the baby teeth begin to appear. The most important function of a good modern dentifrice is to carry topical fluoride. The more often fluoride comes in contact with the tooth, the stronger that tooth is going to be. This is an added surface, or local, protection, and will supplement the fluoride in drinking water, which is doing a different job; it is playing its part in the systemic development of the enamel.

A little bit of dentifrice placed on the gauze that is used to clean the teeth is an excellent way of getting the fluoride onto the tooth. However, for the fluoride to be most effective, the tooth must first be clean and dry. First, take the tooth between the fingers, wipe it carefully to get the film (plaque) off the tooth, and then dry it. Then apply the fluoridated dentifrice to the tooth surface.

Saliva and plaque are protein films that act as barriers against the uptake of fluoride. Placing a fluoride dentifrice on a tooth that has a film of plaque on it is not as effective as placing a fluoride dentifrice on a tooth that has just been cleaned.

You can tell if a commercial dentifrice containing fluoride is reputable by looking on the box for a statement of approval by the Council on Dental Therapeutics of the American Dental Association.

Mouthwashes

For ordinary rinsing, plain water is a terrific mouthwash. I know of no reason for a child to use a commercial mouthwash unless he has some severe caries problem and the mouthwash contains fluoride.

The defenses in a child's mouth are of such a nature that the saliva and the oral bacteria are very effective means of keeping infection out of the mouth. Cuts and bruises within the mouth heal extremely rapidly and, except for lesions such as canker sores, such problems rarely last more than a day or two, at most.

Recent clinical studies with fluoride mouthwashes show extremely promising results. There seems to be good indication that children over three who have caries or continue to show new caries at annual checkups would be well advised to use a fluoride mouthwash after brushing until they bring the caries problem under control.

A word of caution: different fluoride mouthwashes work differently. Some are meant to be swallowed, and some are meant to be swished around and spat out. *Be sure you know which kind your child is using and what he is doing with it.* Fluoride mouthwashes work best when the teeth are clean, just after they have been brushed.

Bad Breath

There is no dental reason for a child with a daily teeth-cleaning routine to have bad breath. Halitosis is much more likely to originate in the stomach or small intestine than in a clean mouth. In an adult, bad breath may be an indication of plaque accumulation, but when a child has bad breath, suspect that some other problem is responsible; it's not coming from the teeth.

A child with bad breath either had garlic for dinner the evening before or is suffering from some gastric or other medical problem, which should be investigated carefully.

TOOTH POSITION AND BAD HABITS

We talk about the primary teeth "erupting" into the mouth, but that is really a rather violent word for the process. It is more of a gliding, sliding movement, with the teeth advancing slowly through the gums, and the gums thinning and parting to allow the advance. There is no such thing as "eruptive force." The "force" that brings a tooth into the mouth is a development of the bone surrounding each individual tooth bud.

If you are watching your child's mouth so that you are aware of the arrival of the primary teeth, and if you're familiar with the chart on page 30, showing the pattern of eruption, then you are probably hoping that your child's teeth are going to line up in an ideal arrangement in the dental arch. However, the position that the tooth assumes in the dental arch is determined by the forces that act on the tooth once it has erupted through the gums. These forces include a number of elements:

- tongue movements that push,
- lip movements that hold in,
- movements of cheek muscles,
- pressure that occurs when the tooth meets an opposing tooth in the other jaw,
- the effect on the tooth of atmospheric pressure every time the child swallows or closes his mouth.

It is possible by examining the position of the teeth in the primary dentition to get a fair idea of the various forces that are going to act on the permanent teeth when they start to erupt into the mouth, about the time the child is six or seven. Forces that push the baby teeth toward faulty closure will probably have to be dealt with in the arrangement of the permanent teeth.

If, when the child closes his jaw, there is a steep overbite (the upper teeth come forward and cover the lower line of teeth), or if the midlines are not parallel when the child closes his jaw (does the gap between the two front top teeth line up with the gap between the two front bottom teeth?), there may be a pernicious habit that is exerting pressure in your child's mouth. Let's describe some of these habits, and then you can check your family out. Are any of these practices showing up in your household?

Many malocclusions are caused by an imbalance in the pressures of the muscle systems that are guiding the teeth into position or holding them in position where they belong. It is possible, when we're made aware of them, to detect the presence of bad habits that create this imbalance before they have an opportunity to affect the developing dentition and before the habits result in a fixed musculature pattern that the child may continue to repeat for the rest of his life.

Lip-sucking, tongue-thrusting, nail-biting, cheek-biting — these are habits that, like thumb- and finger-sucking for infants and toddlers, may serve emotional needs. Try to evaluate the habit before you begin a campaign to get rid of it. Is it a mannerism or positional habit that the child, with encouragement and reminding, is ready to give up? Is it a habit hanging on from early childhood, which new status as a "big kid" will help lay to rest? Or is it a compulsive habit that is connected with some deep emotional need on the child's part?

You may have to decide to let the underlying need express itself in a "bad" habit — even though orthodontic treatment will later be needed to correct the results — on the grounds that crooked teeth are easier to straighten than a warped personality.

If, however, you do decide to work with the child to end a harmful oral habit, you should bear these points in mind:

1. The child must agree on the objective, and want to lose the habit.
2. You must bring the habit to the child's consciousness to make him recognize it. For the first few weeks, every time your child repeats the habit, say, "Hey, what are you doing?"
3. A habit is a repeated muscular activity that is done unconsciously. You break it the same way you begin it — by repetition. The more times a child *does not* perform the habit, the nearer he is to dropping it altogether.

Lip-Biting

One of the earliest and most common of all habits causing malocclusion is that of lip-biting. There is no reason for a well child to have chapped lips, even during the winter. If your child has chapped lips — especially a chapped lower lip — check for lip-biting.

Most parents are unaware that their child is engaging in such a habit. But inspection of a child's lips even when she is as young as two will show a tendency toward lip-biting if it exists: look to see if the red portion of the lower lip is larger than the upper lip. In school a child sitting and biting her lip looks rather thoughtful and studious. We may not recognize this as a pernicious habit at first. In little girls it is often attractive and thought of as a "pouty" look. However, close examination of the vermilion border (the lip line) of the lower lip will show it to be diffuse, with no sharp demarcation between the pink and the red.

Tongue-Thrusting

Tongue-thrusting is another bad habit, one of the most difficult muscular habits the dentist has to deal with. If it could be prevented, most difficult orthodontic cases would be self-correcting.

Bad Habits and How to Detect Them

Lip-biting	Chapped lips; lower lip larger than top
Tongue-thrusting	Muscles over chin wrinkling when child swallows
Nail-biting	No need to cut nails
Cheek-biting	Swollen flap of tissue inside cheek
Finger-biting	Callus on finger
Thumb-sucking	A clean thumb

Observe your child quietly and unobtrusively. If he has a tongue-thrust habit, each time he swallows he will thrust his tongue forward and push it between the upper and lower teeth when they are in occlusion.

I'd almost rather a child sucked his thumb than bit his lower lip. There's a lot of social pressure on a thumb-sucker, from family and peers, that keeps him from exercising the habit all the time, while a lip-biter looks preoccupied, and no one thinks to discourage the habit.

As the lip gets dry from being wet by the tongue, it tends to itch. The child has a tendency to pull it up inside his mouth and scratch it with his upper teeth and then wet it again. As he wets it he takes the oils out of the skin, which dries up and becomes chapped and irritated. The child, then, tends to scratch the lip again with his upper teeth, wet his lip with his tongue, and allow it to dry out. He keeps repeating these actions.

An aid in helping a child break a lip-biting habit is an emollient, such as a Chap Stick, Vaseline, or cold cream, placed on the part of the lip the child bites. This is soothing, and there won't be quite so much urge to scratch the lip because it won't feel dry and itchy. It takes many months to break a habit once it is formed, so it's best to start working on it as soon as the habit is detected. Be aware of the possibility of such habits being formed by your child very early, especially before the third year.

Fingernail-Biting

Many children start to bite on their fingernails when they are as young as two years. Those mothers who find that they never have to cut their children's fingernails may be in the best position to diagnose the habit. Fingernail-biting usually causes the rotations that we see in the teeth in the anterior section of the mouth. It may also contribute to a slight wearing away of the biting surfaces, and of course it introduces germs and dirt into the mouth.

As with any habit, aroused self-awareness, helpful reminders — and, in this case, perhaps social disapproval from peers — contribute to its breaking.

Cheek-Biting

First, look inside the mouth for a swollen flap of skin. Cheek-biting is one of the most difficult habits for parents to detect. Since it occurs only when the teeth are together and the mouth is closed, you'll have to watch for outside signs of interior movement in order to detect the presence of the habit. Point out to the child what he is doing, and help him watch for its recurrence.

Tooth-Grinding

Tooth-grinding (the dental term is "bruxism") probably starts even before the first tooth comes into the mouth. There is a tendency in some children to gnash their upper and lower jaws together while sleeping and sometimes while at rest during the day. It is an expression of a muscular habit that serves as a tension-releasing device. As his teeth start coming into his mouth, the child who is a "bruxist" can make a considerable amount of noise by grinding his teeth when he lies in bed.

Bruxism alone does not cause malocclusion, but it can tend to delay the loss (exfoliation) of the primary teeth. The permanent teeth have a much more difficult time coming into the mouth when bruxism is practiced. The time of their eruption may be delayed, the sequence of eruption is often disturbed, and malocclusion may result from these interferences.

A child who is a confirmed bruxist will probably do little to his primary teeth, with all that grinding, except keep them extremely clean and prevent cavities, since he wears them away faster than they can decay. But he must be watched extremely carefully when it comes time for him to lose his primary teeth. Your dentist may not be aware that your child is a tooth-grinder. Tell him, and be prepared to have some teeth taken out if they do not fall out at the correct time. To my knowledge, there's no known way of breaking the habit of bruxism. Sometimes, when it persists until the child has his or her permanent dentition, it's associated with periodontal disease and jaw problems.

Keeping a Mouthful of Things

Objects such as blanket corners, shoelaces, shirt sleeves, toys, and so forth are used by children as substitutes for their thumb and as pacifiers for biting and chewing. Used for short periods of time, none of these is dangerous. (Think of the substitutes we adults use: cigarettes, cigars, gum, pencils, pipes.) However, when a child keeps one of these in his mouth for many hours a day, malocclusion generally results. It's true that all children should be allowed to bite and chew and suck and to enjoy these oral activities, but they should be discouraged from doing any of these things constantly, hour after hour, day after day.

A Final Word About Pacifiers

In general, I find pacifiers an important outlet. I recommend that parents not do *anything* about them. The energy expended by a child on a pacifier very often finds its expression, when it is displaced, in other more objectionable types of behavior — for example, temper tantrums or bed-wetting. Most children give up the habit when they are subjected to social pressure from their peers, around the age of five or six. They're easier to reason with then, too, but a three-year-old can be dealt with only on an emotional level. That's the time I would become aggressive. Until Linus is three, I believe that he should have his security blanket; I don't believe in taking it away from him.

I do not use mechanical means to *prevent* children from engaging in such habits as thumb-sucking. I will sometimes make them an appliance that acts as a *reminder* not to suck their thumb. It doesn't punish, or even prevent — the thumb just doesn't feel the way it used to. The child generally gives up the habit when he doesn't get the old biofeedback.

REPORT CARD   THREE YEARS

Look for these characteristics in your three-year-old. If you don't answer "yes" to these questions, look back at this section for more information. See page 21 on the best way to examine your child's mouth. Remember, use a good light.

Soft Tissues	Can the child stick his tongue tip completely out of his mouth?
TONGUE	Can he swallow with his teeth together—without the
LIPS	tongue pushing through each time?
CHEEK	Are upper and lower lip the same size?
GUMS	Is the lower lip free of chapping and cracking?
	Is there a clear distinction between lip and skin of face?
	When you look inside cheeks, are the entrances to the parotid glands even in size and not swollen?
	Is the color inside the cheeks even throughout?
	Are gum tissues same color, top and bottom? Front to back? Are gums free of pimples? No swelling? (There should be no swelling, as no teeth are coming through just now.)

Hard Tissues	*Number*
	Are there 20 teeth? Do you find 10 up and 10 down?
	Are there the same number of teeth on either side of the midline?
	Are the teeth on either side of the midline the same shape?
	Bite
	When your child closes his mouth, do the top teeth bite over the bottom teeth?
	Do all the teeth come in contact when jaw is closed?
	Are the teeth spaced out, not crowded?

Color

Are the teeth milky-white?

Are the teeth an even color from tips to gumline?

Are the top, bottom, front, and back teeth all the same color?

Do any stains and colors come off easily with a toothbrush?

Hygiene

Are the teeth clean?

Does the mouth have a clean, sweet odor?

Are *you* still brushing your child's teeth?

REPORT CARD   SIX YEARS

Look for these characteristics in your six-year-old. If you don't answer "yes" to these questions, look back at this section for more information. See page 21 on the best way to examine your child's mouth. Remember, use a good light.

Soft Tissues

TONGUE
LIPS
CHEEK
GUMS

Can the child stick his tongue tip completely out of his mouth? Is tongue free of white coating?

Can he swallow with his teeth together—without the tongue pushing through each time?

Are upper and lower lip the same size?

Is the lower lip free of chapping and cracking?

Is there a clear distinction between lip and skin of face?

When you look inside cheeks, are the entrances to the parotid glands even in size and not swollen?

Is the color inside the cheeks even throughout?

Are gum tissues same color, top and bottom? Front to back? Are gums free of pimples?

Is the tissue between the teeth firm, or loose and puffy? If you press it with your fingertip, does it bleed? (It shouldn't.)

Hard Tissues

Number

How many teeth are there? Are the front top or bottom teeth getting loose?

Have the permanent molars started to come in? Remember, they come in behind, not under, the primary molars.

Bite

When your child closes his mouth, do the top teeth bite over the bottom teeth?

Do all the teeth come in contact when jaw is closed?

Are the teeth spaced out, not crowded?

Are you and your child pleased with the appearance of the teeth?

Color

Are the teeth milky-white?

Are the teeth an even color from tips to gumline?

Are the top, bottom, front, and back teeth all the same color?

Do any stains and colors come off easily with a toothbrush?

Hygiene

Are the teeth clean?

Does the mouth have a clean, sweet odor?

Do you check each day that the brushing has been done?

Does your child use disclosing tablets?

REPORT CARD   NINE YEARS

Look for these characteristics in your nine-year-old. If you don't answer "yes" to these questions, look back at this section for more information. See page 21 on the best way to examine your child's mouth. Remember, use a good light.

Soft tissues

TONGUE
LIPS
CHEEK
GUMS

Can the child stick his tongue tip completely out of his mouth? Is tongue free from white coating?

Can he swallow with his teeth together—without the tongue pushing through each time?

Are upper and lower lip the same size?

Is the lower lip free of chapping and cracking?

Is there a clear distinction between lip and skin of face?

When you look inside cheeks, are the entrances to the parotid glands even in size and not swollen?

Is the color inside the cheeks even throughout?

Are gum tissues same color, top and bottom? Front to back? Are gums free of pimples? Push the tongue aside and check the tongue side of the gum for abscesses.

Is the tissue between the teeth firm, or loose and puffy? If you press it with your fingertip, does it bleed? (It shouldn't.)

Hard Tissues	*Number*

How many teeth are there? There should now be at least four front permanent teeth in the upper and lower jaws, and four permanent molars, two up and two down.

Bite

When your child closes his mouth, do the top teeth bite over the bottom teeth?

Do all the teeth come in contact when jaw is closed?

Are the teeth spaced out, not crowded?

Are the remaining primary molars worn down—is there any sign of grinding (brusixm)?

Are all the teeth at the same height in the jaw?

Are you and your child pleased with the appearance of the teeth?

Color

The permanent teeth are a shade darker than the primary teeth; are the new permanent teeth ivory-colored and evenly shaded throughout?

Are the top, bottom, front and back teeth all the same color?

Do any stains and colors come off easily with a toothbrush?

Hygiene

Are the teeth clean?

Does the mouth have a clean, sweet odor?

Is your child using disclosing tablets?

Is your child flossing in addition to brushing?

Does he have two toothbrushes? (It takes a day for one to dry out.)

Has he had a new toothbrush in the last 6 months?

REPORT CARD   TWELVE YEARS

Look for these characteristics in your twelve-year-old. If you don't answer
"yes" to these questions, look back at this section for more information. See
page 21 on the best way to examine your child's mouth. Remember, use a
good light.

Soft Tissues   Can the child stick his tongue tip completely out of his
                  mouth? Is tongue free of white coating?
TONGUE   Can he swallow with his teeth together—without the
LIPS   tongue pushing through each time?
CHEEK   Are upper and lower lip the same size?
GUMS   Is the lower lip free of chapping and cracking?
                  Is there a clear distinction between lip and skin of face?
                  When you look inside cheeks, are the entrances to the
                    parotid glands even in size and not swollen?
                  Is the color inside the cheeks even throughout?
                  Are gum tissues same color, top and bottom? Front to
                    back? Are gums free of pimples? Push the tongue aside
                    and check the tongue side of the gum for abscesses.
                  Is the tissue between the teeth firm, or loose and puffy? If
                    you press it with your fingertip, does it bleed? (It
                    shouldn't.)

Hard Tissues   *Number*
                  How many teeth are there?
                  Are there an even number of teeth on either side of the
                    midline?
                  Most of the remaining primary teeth should be getting
                    loose.
                  The upper cuspids (the pointed teeth) should be coming
                    into the mouth.

                  Bite
                  When your child closes his mouth, do the top teeth bite
                    over the bottom teeth?
                  Do all the teeth come in contact when jaw is closed?
                  Do teeth in front look long? When child fails to brush,
                    gum recedes, giving "long-toothed" look.
                  Are you and your child pleased with the appearance of the
                    teeth?

                  Color
                  The permanent teeth are a shade darker than the primary
                    teeth; are the new permanent teeth ivory-colored and
                    evenly shaded throughout?

Are the top, bottom, front, and back teeth all the same color?

Do any stains and colors come off easily with a toothbrush?

Hygiene   Are the teeth clean?

Does the mouth have a clean, sweet odor?

Does the child brush twice a day, floss once?

Does he use disclosing tablets once a week?

Does he have two toothbrushes? (It takes a day for one to dry out.)

Has he had a new toothbrush in the last 6 months?

SPEECH AND TEETH

For many years dentists and speech pathologists felt that the teeth were essential in helping the child speak and pronounce word sounds. A child who lisped or had trouble with his dental sounds — d's, t's — was thought to be having trouble with his teeth. Parents have come to my office to ask if teeth are related to some speech problem their child is having.

To my knowledge, there does not seem to be such a relationship. If a youngster at the age of four or five loses his four primary incisors because of a fall, or has to have them extracted for some reason, his speech pattern does indeed change — for two or three weeks. After that, he sounds exactly as he did before.

The same thing happens when a child wears an appliance. If a dentist makes an appliance for a child to remind him to stop sucking his thumb or to move anterior teeth back, the child's speech pattern alters for a couple of days; then the child's mouth adjusts and the speech returns to normal.

I think most speech problems are not tooth-related. I think it's what the child hears, in addition to a combination of muscular movements. I have seen children recommended for orthodontics when speech pathologists became frustrated and hoped that changing the position of the tongue or tooth or lip was going to solve their problem. I wish a dentist could help in this area, but I just think the answer is not in our hands.

CLEANING TECHNIQUES AS YOUR CHILD GROWS OLDER
(See also pages 87–91)

Toothbrushes

As the molars start to come into the mouth, cleaning the little grooves and crevices on the surfaces of the molar teeth is too difficult a job for the little square of gauze to do, so when the child is around two or two and a half, the mother or father should start using a toothbrush in the child's mouth. It really doesn't matter whether you use a nylon- or a natural-bristle toothbrush with a child. The objective is getting the crumbs and plaque off the teeth. A brush with a small head, a straight handle, and a flat brushing surface is fine. It's a good idea to have two brushes, so that one is always dry and ready for use.

If one parent has been spending time cleaning the child's mouth and watching the teeth come into the mouth, he or she will know when they are dirty. It is still necessary, until the child is around five, to brush her teeth twice a day — after breakfast and after the last meal in the evening. Perhaps parents would like to alternate the duty, with one taking the responsibility in the morning and the other in the evening, as it fits their schedules.

Another good use of the toothbrush is for brushing the top surface of the tongue. The top of the tongue is covered with the same tissue as that which covers the teeth and gum pads — literally, the skin of your teeth. Brushing the tongue once in a while is a great help in reducing the number of oral bacteria and plaque-forming organisms.

In spite of their encouragement to a child to use a toothbrush alone, parents must remember that it is their responsibility to keep the child's teeth clean. It's particularly hard for a young child to clean the back teeth. The best way to reach these teeth is for the parent to cradle child's head in the crook of her arm while she makes a back-and-forth brushing stroke on the biting surfaces of the child's teeth, followed by a whisking up-and-down stroke on the tongue and on the cheek sides. Look at the illustration on page 20, showing how to examine your child's teeth. This position is good for toothbrushing, too.

Cleaning the primary teeth with a toothbrush can best be described as a scrub technique. Any motion that will get the food and debris off the top and sides of the tooth with a toothbrush is an acceptable method. Since children, by and large, do not have gum disease, intricate instructions for placing the brush or moving it are not necessary for cleaning the primary dentition. (A soft-scrub technique that a child can master is described step-by-step on pages 82–83.) An electric toothbrush, when used correctly, is more efficient in cleaning the teeth than a standard toothbrush. However, a child who is not in the habit of having a standard toothbrush used in his mouth will not allow the invasion of an electric toothbrush.

Many parents purchase electric toothbrushes for their children in the hope that they will use them, but in a few days the novelty wears off. If the child does not have the habit of brushing his teeth routinely with a regular brush, he is not going to be able to make the transition to the electric model, and parents who hope their children will are only deluding themselves.

Old Wives' Tale

"A strong antiseptic mouthwash will destroy bacteria that cause decay."

Even the most effective commercial mouthwash will reduce the number of bacteria in the mouth for only a matter of minutes. If you used one strong enough to destroy all the bacteria, you would damage the delicate tissues of your mouth. It's better to think of a mouthwash as a pleasant-tasting rinse that gets rid of food particles loosened by your brush — and not as a means for killing bacteria.

Mouthwashes

No evidence exists that the routine use of a mouthwash will cut down on the number of colds a child has or that it will be at all beneficial in helping the child recover from a cold that he may have at the time. Using a mouthwash does not — repeat, does not — remove food particles from between the teeth. Nor does it eliminate bad breath; it only masks it, just as a flavored dentifrice does, for short periods of time.

The new fluoride mouthwashes do one thing: they bring fluoride in contact with the tooth. If your child uses one, he should do so at the end of the cleaning routine.

Toothpastes

A dentifrice acts primarily as a carrier for detergent and for fluoride. Many people go merrily through life without ever using one. This is certainly permissible. Salt and water or baking soda and water are also excellent for cleaning the teeth. Many individuals choose to brush their teeth with water and nothing else. The object, after all, is removal of debris from the teeth.

If a fluoride dentifrice is not used you must be careful to get topical fluoride on the teeth in other ways. The use of a topical fluoride gel, applied during routine visits to the dentist, is one way to get topical fluoride, but you can't do that every day. It's safe to use a topical fluoride even when your local water supply is fluoridated; you're not going to overdo it.

Water-Irrigating Devices

Water-irrigating devices (Water Pik is one brand) are a lot of fun. Functionally, they are excellent tools for wetting the bathroom floor, the bathroom mirror, and pajamas. They are useful, too, for older people who have braces, bridges, and other equipment in their mouths.

Because you find that a water jet feels good, you can't understand why everybody shouldn't use one. But you are a grown-up, dealing, perhaps, with gum problems as well as bridges and caps. Children don't get the same physical sensation because they don't have the same situation.

Water jets do little to remove dental plaque from teeth. Primary teeth and young permanent teeth generally have spaces between them and do not collect food, so the use of a water-irrigating device to remove particles of food is of little value in children. Teen-agers may find these devices helpful in cleaning their wisdom teeth (see page 64).

Dental Floss

It is difficult, if not impossible, to reach the plaque in between all teeth at all times with the aid of a toothbrush. The only way to clean in between the teeth adequately is by rubbing or buffing those areas with a piece of dental floss. By shining the neighboring surfaces of each tooth with dental floss, you'll be able to remove the plaque, bacteria, and food that harbor there and prevent the caries that form between these teeth. It's a good idea to practice flossing at least once a day.

In a child, there are four spots that need regular flossing. They are between the last two molars on each side of each jaw. Try to make flossing these four sites part of the evening cleaning routine. Again, you'll have to do it until your child can handle it alone. (See pages 85–86 for proper flossing technique.)

GREEN, BLACK, ORANGE STAINS

Inside, outside: green, black, orange. At different intervals in the developing dentition, a child's teeth may develop strange colors.

Tetracycline Stain

In the late 1950s and early sixties, the drug tetracycline was a popular antibiotic for children and adults. Physicians and pediatricians used it for infections, especially for those accompanied by fevers. The problem: tetracycline is a dye; it will stain any tissue that is mineralizing at the time of its use. If a pregnant woman takes it, it will stain the teeth that are forming in the baby in utero. After birth, the child's primary teeth will often be found to look yellow or orange.

Some very young children who were given the drug between birth and five years had their developing permanent teeth stained. Today their teeth are dark gray to yellow to orange.

What can be done about it?

Now that we know what the effects are, we don't give pregnant women and children this drug. There are other antibiotics available. Most pediatricians know this, but it doesn't hurt for parents to ask what drug is being given their child. You may have a pediatrician who got his or her training in the fifties and thinks of tetracycline as a reliable drug that has worked in the past.

A tooth that has within it a green, yellow, or orange cast is considered a tetracycline-stained tooth. To identify such teeth, look at a history of medications the child has been given, and test the teeth by shining an ultraviolet light on them. They will give a greenish-orange glow if the stain was caused by tetracycline.

The old treatment was to bleach the teeth over a period of months with a peroxide solution and strong light. This is ineffective: it doesn't last.

I prefer a new dental material, a liquid quartz that can be painted over the teeth, and caused to harden. This gives a natural color to the teeth. And newer dental materials for this purpose will be discovered in the future. (See the illustration on page 94.)

Green Stain

Green teeth usually occur in the upper jaw in the front of the mouth at the gum line. This condition is caused by plants called algae — the same algae you find in your fish tank. They grow only where there is light — that is, in the front of the mouth, on the top front teeth — and they grow at the gum line, where the climate is moist and they can obtain food. Parents can remove the green stain at home by taking a piece of gauze, placing a little dentifrice on it, and scrubbing away just where the tooth meets the gum line. The green color doesn't mean the teeth are impaired, but it does make the teeth look odd.

Black Stain

Black stain (sometimes called "pellicle") develops in a number of children. You'll notice it, if it exists, as dark, black lines running along the gum line of most of the teeth. It forms when the surface of the tooth becomes stained by some of the salts that occur naturally in the saliva. It is difficult to remove by mechanical means — that is, with a toothbrush or a piece gauze and dentifrice. It can be removed in a dentist's office with a rotating rubber polishing cup. However, it re-forms rather quickly. Pellicle tends to disappear as the permanent teeth come into the mouth and the child reaches nine or ten years of age. If your child has this stain, in some ways he is lucky, for children who have pellicle tend to develop few dental cavities. Exactly what the relationship is between pellicle and dental cavities nobody yet knows.

Orange Stain

Orange stain is usually found at the gum line in upper and lower teeth. It is caused by color-producing (chromogenic) bacteria. Why some children have these orange-colored bacteria and some don't have them is not known. It is thought that children who drink a lot of milk tend to grow the golden- or orange-colored bacteria. This stain, too, can be removed at home with a gauze pad and a little bit of dentifrice rubbed vigorously at the gum line. Children with chromogenic bacteria are often very susceptible to dental caries. If your child has a colony of "orange bugs" growing on his front teeth, it usually means that somebody is falling down on the job of cleaning the child's teeth.

Very white teeth are not necessarily healthy teeth. Your child's adult teeth may come through looking much yellower than the milky-white baby teeth, or they may have an ivory cast. This is natural, in spite of the movie-star flash of white we are conditioned to admire. In fact, whiteness may indicate a soft, porous enamel.

THE MOST IMPORTANT TEETH

When the child is about six, the first permanent tooth arrives in the mouth: the six-year molar. Because it does not replace a lost baby tooth but comes in behind the second baby molar, some parents do not realize that it's a permanent tooth. But you'll know because you've been checking and counting and familiarizing yourself with your child's first set of teeth.

If there has been no premature loss of baby teeth, the six-year molars will come into the mouth in place. (One of the jobs baby teeth perform is stabilizing the position of permanent teeth.) These six-year molars are probably the most important teeth in the mouth. If they are in their proper place, they act as foundations for the dental arch and keep all the other teeth in their proper positions. A dentist can often take a look at the way the six-year molars fit in the arch and predict whether occlusion is going to be normal or not.

When these four new permanent teeth are in place, each in its corner of the jaws, they hold the jaws in position in relation to each other while the primary teeth are being shed — another example of nature's timing. While holding this height as the primary teeth in front are being lost, they also serve as natural space maintainers for the permanent second (twelve-year) molars that will come in behind them.

If any teeth in the mouth are to be guarded and protected, it is these teeth. If a cavity occurs, it should be promptly filled. And I can hardly imagine a situation in which a six-year molar should be extracted. Such a step can lead to complex and expensive orthodontic corrections or permanent problems in the position and fit of the teeth. Cherish that tooth! Many dentists are placing a plastic sealant on the biting surface of the six-year molar as added insurance against its getting a cavity (see page 93).

WHAT TO DO ABOUT A LOOSE PRIMARY TOOTH

When primary teeth become loose, they will often hang around in front or back for weeks at a time, and become painful to chew on and irritating to the gums. Parents are at a loss to know what to do.

My advice is, just take the tooth between two fingers, give it a sharp tug, and take it out. There's probably little pain in this quick yank — no more than in pulling out a single hair — a short sensation, soon gone. The pain was from the loose tooth's being pushed against soft tissue. If any bleeding occurs afterward, it can be controlled with pressure. Hold a little piece of cotton or gauze on the gum for a few minutes.

Parents come into my office with a child who has had a loose primary tooth for a week or two; the gum is sore and inflamed. But there's no need to wait that long. Be brave; go ahead and pull it. If it's not loose enough, it won't come out. If you really want to let the dentist do the job for you on a stubborn tooth, he will. He'll flow a few drops of an anesthetic solution directly next to the tooth and then lift it out with no pain to the child.

If a loose primary tooth inadvertently gets swallowed, don't worry. The enamel will not be digested. And the tooth is small — it will pass right through the digestive tract like a seed or cherry pit. Children swallow things like that all the time.

Old Wives' Tale

"When a child loses a primary tooth, the Tooth Fairy comes at night and takes the tooth from under the pillow, leaving a coin in its place."

True. This has happened in experiment after experiment, in generations of families. Dentists are at a loss to explain this scientifically, but reassure their patients that anything that makes losing primary teeth a little more fun is dentally okay.

INJURIES AND TRAUMAS

I suppose one of the most upsetting things — to parent and child — is an accident in which a child's tooth is fractured or knocked out. It's painful for the child and an emergency situation for the parent.

The majority of these injuries result from simple accidents — minor falls, sports mishaps, childish pranks. As you may guess, they most often involve the front teeth, so in addition to pain and discomfort, there's the problem of appearance.

Although many accidents befall the toddler, statistics show that children aged nine and ten are the most susceptible to damage, and boys are about twice as likely as girls to have such an accident.

Try to remember to fasten seat belts in your automobile to avoid injury to the face, head, and teeth, and have your child wear a mouth guard when he or she participates in contact sports.

Care of Injuries

Sometimes a fall or other injury will knock a tooth out completely. The best thing to do is to wipe the tooth free of dirt (rinse under cold water if necessary) and stick it firmly back in the socket — as far as it will go. Some parents can't bring themselves to do this, but if the tooth isn't back in the mouth within, at most, twenty minutes, the chance of successful reimplantation diminishes rapidly. Since every playground, schoolyard, and swimming pool is not equipped with a dentist, you might be called on to perform such first aid.

Even if the tooth isn't back in place within twenty minutes, all is not lost. Get the tooth (which should be kept damp) and child to a dentist or to a hospital or medical center emergency room with a dentist on duty. Depending on the condition of the tooth and child, he will replace the tooth in the mouth. Sometimes a reimplanted tooth will give years' more service. If a reimplanted primary tooth lasts one to three years, that's all the time you need before the underlying permanent tooth is ready to take its place. If the reimplanted tooth is a permanent one, then in about the same time as the tooth will begin to die, the root will resorb, and the tooth will loosen and fall out. No one has figured out how to arrest the process, although many — including me — are trying different implantation techniques.

The best way to transport a tooth that has been knocked out of a child's mouth to a dentist is to have the child hold the tooth in his mouth under his tongue until the dentist places it back in its correct position. The saliva in the mouth provides the best emergency environment.

In an accident that results in a fractured or chipped tooth in which the nerve is not exposed, wipe the tooth with warm water, keep it clean, and as soon as possible get to a dentist so that he or she can place a covering over the exposed dentin and give the tooth time to heal.

With fractured permanent teeth, there have been amazing advances in repair. In the past, a dentist would cut the tooth down and put a cap on it. Today, there are tooth-colored materials that can be bonded directly to the tooth, without the use of anesthesia and without any cutting of the tooth structure. It is liquid quartz, the same material used to fix teeth with stains caused by tetracycline. Many young people who have chips and cracks in their front teeth and didn't want, or couldn't afford, caps are being treated with this material. I see many teen-agers in my office who have spent six or seven self-conscious years, and in just one visit walk out with a restoration that is indistinguishable from a natural, whole tooth.

PROTECTING TEETH AT SCHOOL AND AT PLAY

All along the way there are hazards to teeth from injury or accident. The toddler falls down in the course of learning to walk and run; the three-year-old has blocks and swings and tricycles to contend with; and just as the older child begins to get a mouthful of permanent teeth, he or she goes in for a competitive sport and begins to use new tools and machines, such as bicycles and skateboards, for individual play.

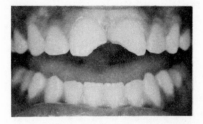
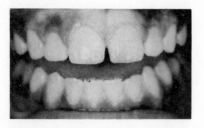

While playing hockey this twelve-year-old boy fractured his upper two central incisors. Fortunately the nerves of the teeth were not exposed, and his dentist was able to bond the plastic directly to the teeth. It is almost impossible to distinguish the repaired teeth from the original.

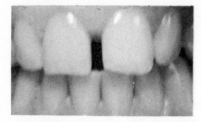
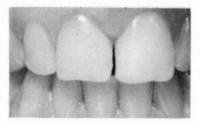

This fourteen-year-old girl was unhappy about the large space between her upper two front teeth. Her dentist added a bit of the new material to each tooth. She was pleased with her smile.

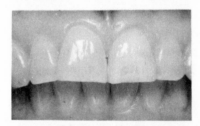
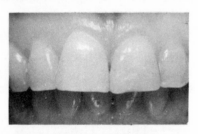

The left central incisor in the mouth of this ten-year-old erupted with a yellow spot on its front surface. By using the new material, the child's dentist was able to make the tooth look natural.

ESTHETICS FOR CHILDREN

These before-and-after photographs illustrate the use of a new dental material that enables dentists to restore and reshape front teeth without cutting the tooth to make room for a filling material or a cap. The material is a tooth-colored plastic that can be bonded directly to the tooth.

Safety education is important for dental health. Here are some areas in which a child can be instructed. The school is probably emphasizing the same things.*

Football	Wear properly fitted mouth guard and helmet.
Baseball	Wear catcher's mask when receiving pitched balls.
Basketball	Wear a mouth guard, especially in rough games.
Boxing	Always wear a mouth guard.
Running Games	Never trip or upset another player during play. Don't carry dangerous objects when you run.
Riding in Cars	Be aware of sudden stops. Use a seat belt.
Swimming and Diving	Use the ladder to climb out of the pool. Don't run or push when near a pool.
Tree-Climbing	Never climb a wet tree. Be sure of your footing.
Bicycling	Obey all traffic laws. Be careful in rainy weather. Wet roads and wet leaves make biking very dangerous.
Ice-Skating	Don't push or trip other skaters. Wear a mouth guard when playing hockey.
Roller-Skating	Don't go too fast. Keep skates under control. Never "hitch" rides.
Swinging	Remain seated. Don't jump from or walk under a moving swing.
Sledding	Watch out for trees and other obstacles in your path.
Skateboarding	Apply nonskid tape to top of skateboard. Avoid busy streets and sidewalks. Avoid slopes — look for a flat surface.
Drinking Fountains	Don't say "Hi" to friends when they're drinking at fountains.

*Adapted from the Detroit District Dental Society.

TEETH AND TEEN-AGERS

There comes a time in the lives of parents when they look at their children and wonder, "Where did they come from — these strange, tall children, living in our home like boarders who don't pay rent and can't be evicted? Can these be the same children who twelve years ago were so charming and bright?" When we welcomed these babies with open arms, did we really understand that they would someday turn into teen-agers?

It's hard for a teen-ager to find a dentist he or she can trust. Until they have the security of knowing where they are themselves, teen-agers find dentists psychologically threatening. Their reluctance to have their mouths "invaded" is a displaced sexual fear.

I feel that the best way to reach teen-age patients is to try to establish and maintain a strong personal relationship with them. Speak to your teen-agers maturely and honestly. Tell them that it will make you happy and make them happy if they take care of their teeth.

There's not a teen-ager alive who is not thinking about sex . . . how he appears to others, how he smiles, how his breath smells. Self-concepts and esthetics are strong motivating factors during the teens.

Get across to your teen-ager some positive message: "It makes you look brighter . . . Your smile looks good . . . It brightens up your face." These are encouraging words for teen-agers.

Young people are not, as a rule, future-oriented; it does little good to talk to them about dental troubles they may face in their twenties and thirties.

As a dentist, I prefer to talk to a teen-ager without a parent around. I say to her, "Look, it's up to you. Your mother and your father have nothing to do with it anymore. You take care of your teeth or you don't. You know what's going on in your mouth. It's something you have to take care of for yourself."

She also needs consistent and constant home and peer pressure. I know that parents don't like to hear this, but if Mom and Dad don't set a good example — if they are not committed to a self-care routine themselves — the child knows it and thinks of the parents as hypocritical. Advice and warnings then don't have any effect.

Bad Breath and Bleeding Gums

A boy or girl of thirteen can understand scientifically that the odor from his or her mouth is from gas given off by the activity of the bacteria that live there. It is not caused by food sitting around in the mouth for too long. It is gas — hydrogen sulfide — the same gas that comes out of sewers. The only way to get rid of it is by daily cleaning.

It's ironic that just when teen-agers become more aware of their looks, they become more careless of their diet and oral hygiene. Teen-agers will try candy mints, chewing gum, mouthwashes, and other advertised products to sweeten their breath, and will neglect the one sure thing: vigorous brushing and flossing. To show them what they're *actually* doing with their cleaning routine, suggest that they use a plaque-disclosing tablet once a week (see pages 90–91).

The search for movie-star teeth may lead to the use of an abrasive dentifrice or one containing strong bleaches. Try to steer your teen-agers away from these products without making them feel foolish.

Teen-agers sometimes experience tender, bleeding gums, and their first thought is to stay away from the troublesome area. Actually, the very opposite treatment is called for: the more they brush and floss, the sooner the condition will clear up.

Smoking

The teen years are a time of experimentation. This may lead to smoking, a habit that affects the teeth, palate, tongue, gums, lips, and throat, not to mention the total health of an individual. We know this now to be a scientific fact. It is a responsibility for all of us to dissuade teen-agers from beginning to smoke. Again, be factual and forthright with your child: smokers have more gum disease, more oral cancer, stained teeth, bad breath, and deadened palates.

Teen-Age Orthodontics

The teen years are not too late for orthodontics. If your child has a problem in occlusion, orthodontics can correct it. But in the teen years it will be more important than ever to accompany orthodontic treatment with careful cleaning and good nutrition.

Wisdom Teeth

Wisdom teeth — actually, third molars — usually come into the mouth in the late teens. Often a wisdom tooth is impacted — stuck against the molar in front of it — and must be removed. X-rays will have shown the dentist whether the third molars are erupting in the right position and whether there is going to be room for these last molars in the dental arch.

All third molars don't have to be removed. Most discomfort comes from poor oral hygiene; they are difficult teeth to clean. If you'd like to try retaining those teeth, you may find that a water-irrigating device and strenuous brushing does the job.

Teen-Age Diets

Some teen-agers eat the worst food of any people, and the reason is not poverty. The potato-chip-and-cola diet many teen-agers become addicted to can be blamed on numerous elements. Many families no longer eat meals together as the children grow older, and children are allowed to raid the refrigerator and forage for themselves. Teen-agers develop food fads and food preferences that limit their diets. They eat what their friends at the corner snack bar eat. Lots of sugars and carbohydrates are consumed in an effort to provide quick energy for sports and other strenuous activities and to face situations of emotional stress.

Not only do teen-agers eat nutritionless food, but they eat many times a day, a habit that feeds the bacteria as well as the teen-ager. Studies show that the average teen-ager eats nine times a day — usually snack foods, filled with sugar. Snacks are a way of life for many teen-agers; part of their social pattern.

All of this can add up to rampant dental decay. Even if careful diet and regular dental care were part of early childhood, the effects can be wiped out by neglect and bad habits during the adolescent years.

So much is going on in the lives of these young people — physical, emotional, and social changes — that much of the resulting stress shows up in their general health, specifically in the teeth. Let's not give up our ambition — good teeth for our children's lifetime — at this vulnerable time in their lives.

Important Milestones in the Growth and Development of Your Child's Dentition

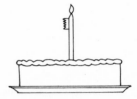

By the first birthday, the bottom and top front teeth have come through the gum and into the mouth, even though the roots are not yet fully formed. The first primary molars are about to appear, and beneath the gums the crowns of the second primary molars are fully formed. Deep in the jaw, the biting surfaces of the first permanent molars are complete, and the first permanent incisors are hardening. The jaw increases in height and width as the cartilage and bone of the jaw grow.

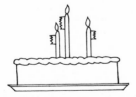

By the time the child is three years old, all twenty primary teeth are generally present and accounted for, and occlusion (the way the teeth fit together) is being established. Beneath the gums, the crowns of the permanent incisors are almost complete; the permanent canines are about two thirds complete; and the mineralization of the premolars has just begun. The crowns of the first permanent molars are practically complete; they will slowly rotate forward to face the direction in which they will move through the gums. The roots of all the baby teeth are complete; their pulp chambers are large and the root canals are mature.

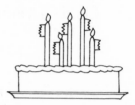

Your five-year-old laughs and shows a row of small, white, evenly spaced teeth. Backstage, a lot is going on. Resorption of the roots of the incisors is beginning; by the time the incisors loosen and fall out, you'll think these teeth didn't have roots at all, but they did. Now they've been resorbed (resorption is like melting) into the tissue of the gums. That's why the primary teeth fall out so easily when the time comes. The roots of the five-year-old's permanent incisors are beginning to mineralize, as are the roots of the first permanent molars.

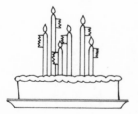 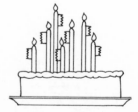

First-graders are in for a lot of firsts, among them the first loose tooth and the first smile with a hole in it. By the time the child is six years of age, x-rays show that the first permanent molars have rapidly developed and moved up behind the primary molars, their roots more than half formed, and the second permanent molars are moving into position. I find that the first permanent molars are often the first permanent teeth to erupt. Usually parents are not aware that their children already have permanent teeth because they tend to erupt without any discomfort.

The front teeth are lost at about this time. The new, permanent incisors grow through the gum. The permanent canines, lying deeper in the jaws, now have fully formed crowns, and the roots of the other primary teeth continue to be resorbed.

Also at this time, growth in the skull and the upper part of the face is nearly finished, but growth in the lower part of the face is still far from complete. The planes of the face are beginning to take on different dimensions, and your first-grader loses his or her "baby face."

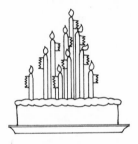

The most dramatic changes in dentition have taken place by the time the child is ten. The permanent incisors are fully in. The primary molars are falling out, one by one, and one or more permanent molars are in place. The latecomers — the canines — are undergoing root resorption, and root formation in the permanent canines is taking place. The second permanent molars are ready to come in, and the third molars (the wisdom teeth) are mineralizing. Parents of children who are nine to thirteen years of age are often concerned about the spaces between their children's upper front teeth — so concerned, in fact, that they seek orthodontic help. It may be useful to know that these spaces don't close naturally until the canine teeth erupt and come into occlusion. When they erupt, two out of three youngsters lose the extra space between their top front teeth naturally.

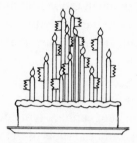

When the child is thirteen, the first and second molars and the canines are in, and the third molars are developing but still under the gum. Except for these last molars, the second dentition — the set of adult teeth — is complete. The muscles of the mouth and face are growing in order to do the work that will be demanded of them by the adult teeth, and the bones of the face and jaw are reaching adult dimensions and strength. And there are thirty-two teeth, ready for a lifetime of use.

PART II

KEYS TO
DEFENSIVE DENTISTRY

THREE

The Anatomy of a Tooth

During the life of the embryo, the cells that are going to manufacture the teeth are beginning to perform their function. Even as early as seven weeks after conception, the cells that will become the tissues of the tooth are already taking form.

HOW A TOOTH BEGINS

The loop of oral epithelium (the thin sheet of closely arranged cells covering the body surface) intrudes into the dental lamina (layer) and begins to distinguish itself as a tooth-forming organ. The upper cells secrete and lay down enamel, which will be the outside of the tooth. The lower cells secrete the dentin, and what is left of the embryonic tissue becomes the pulp cavity. Inside and outside, the tooth cells are being laid down for all twenty primary teeth. Mineralization begins about three months after conception. At birth, most of the baby teeth have mineralized, and beneath them in the jaw the permanent teeth are forming.

Teeth are formed primarily from calcium and phosphate, which are taken from the bloodstream of the mother. She has incorporated these elements into her diet. Vitamin D and thyroid and growth hormones also play a part in the process. When the metabolic factors are normal, the manufacture of the teeth proceeds automatically, and the enamel and dentin crystals are healthy. If the metabolism is not normal, the crystals will mineralize imperfectly.

Although a pregnant mother's diet will affect the whole child, the developing teeth appear to be affected most by an imbalance of calcium and phosphorous salts in the bloodstream. An imbalance in these salts occurs most often from a high fever or a viral infection, not from a nutritional lack.

During tooth formation, the enamel crown forms from different centers on each tooth. Then these centers flow into each other and fuse together. The planes in which they fuse are the grooves and lines you see on the biting surface of molars.

Sometimes the centers don't fuse completely. This leaves a minute opening in the tooth — just big enough for bacteria to fit in. These spaces are called "pits" and "fissures," and they are what the dentist is looking for when he moves his explorer (pick) over the surface of the tooth.

THE PARTS OF A TOOTH

Let's take a look at a tooth — any tooth will do. The part you can see is the *crown;* the part that disappears into and is surrounded by the gum is called the *neck;* and the part you can't see, buried in the bony socket of the jaw and firmly anchored there by soft connecting tissues, is the *root.*

THE SUBSTANCES OF A TOOTH

Enamel

The crown — the visible portion of the tooth — is covered with enamel, the hardest tissue in the body and one of the hardest natural substances known. Its hardness protects it from wear. And yet, hard as it is, it is also vulnerable. Unlike a broken bone, which will heal, a broken, traumatized, or decayed tooth cannot repair itself. It has no contact with the blood, which supplies nutrients to other parts of the body; and since it has no circulatory system, it has no repair cells busily shoring up defenses.

Enamel is composed of small crystals of calcium and phosphate precipitated in a fine matrix of strong protein fibers. Enamel has to be very hard to do the job it is intended to do. First, it has to be resistant to acids, enzymes, and other corrosive substances that are found in the mouth. Then, it must protect the more sensitive tissues in the inner part of the tooth. When you learn that the biting force of chewing can exert 50 to 100 pounds of pressure between the front teeth and 150 to 200 pounds between the teeth in the back, you can see that the enamel must absorb — and protect the dentin and pulp from — this impact.

Enamel is a crystal, and in the mouth it picks up and incorporates various minerals that make it harder. The longer enamel stays in a human's mouth, the harder it gets. That's probably one of the reasons that people over twenty get very few dental caries.

Enamel is also a unique crystal in that it can maintain its hardness over a wide range of temperature changes. It doesn't crack if you follow up ice cream with hot coffee.

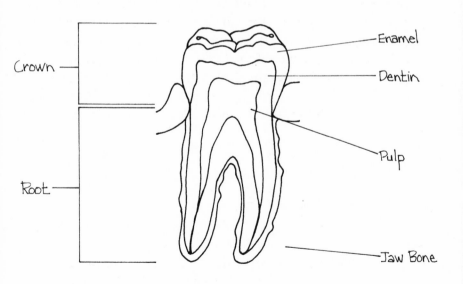

CROSS-SECTION OF A MOLAR TOOTH

Old Wives' Tale

"My children need lots of dental work because they had soft teeth to begin with."

Not true. All teeth are very hard. As a matter of fact, tooth enamel is one of the hardest natural substances there is (diamonds are the hardest). Tooth enamel is much harder than iron, gold, or porcelain. Some teeth are more susceptible to decay than others, but it is never because the teeth are soft. It is because they mineralized imperfectly or were not cared for after they came into the mouth.

Dentin

Dentin is the yellowish, bonelike tissue that lies just under the enamel. It is not as hard as enamel (which is why it needs the enamel to protect it), but is made of essentially the same materials — calcium salts and phosphate embedded in a strong network of protein fibers. Dentin is the bulk of the tooth; the amount of dentin in a tooth determines its size and shape. Fibers from the pulp extend in small canals into the dentin and nourish it. If caries progresses toward the center of the tooth, the dentin cells in the pulp lay down a layer of protective dentin. Unfortunately, this is only a temporary defense, for if left alone, the decay progresses faster than the dentin is laid down, the pulp is invaded, and the tooth loses the battle.

Pulp

When your child has a toothache, the pulp is the part of the tooth that is sending the message. Dental pulp is the soft tissue that fills the chamber at the center of the tooth and the canals that extend down the roots of the tooth. The soft tissue here contains nerves, blood cells, and lymph vessels, and it is the source of the dentin's nutrition and the tooth's communication with the rest of the body. Pain is no fun, but it is the necessary signal to summon defense

Toothache: Emergency Treatment

There are two kinds of toothache generally seen in children, and understanding what causes both will make you better prepared to give first aid.

First is the kind of toothache that occurs while the child is eating something sweet or within a half hour or so after a meal or snack. The child will complain of sharp pain in the tooth. Sugar from the food is in a cavity, feeding the bacteria living at the base of the cavity; the bacteria are producing acid; the acid is burning through the bottom of the tooth, reaching the nerve of the tooth, and causing intense pain.

Put the child down, with head in the examining position (see page 19) in your lap, and find out which tooth is bothering him. Take a toothbrush or toothpick and clean the tooth very aggressively. If you are able to clean out all the food and bacteria this way, then in about fifteen minutes the toothache will disappear. By all means, get him to a dentist right away. Don't wait for another toothache. Decay progresses rapidly in a child's tooth.

The second type of toothache occurs at night and doesn't go away. The tooth is extremely sensitive to touch or to biting down, and the pain is accompanied by a swollen area around the tooth or a swollen jaw and face.

When this happens, it means that decay has progressed and the nerve inside the tooth has died and become infected and abscessed. This is a much more difficult kind of pain to relieve at home. Again, cleaning the tooth quite vigorously is the best thing you can do. See if you can open up the cavity and get out all the food.

Aspirin (swallowed, not held against the tooth) will relieve pain, but the only real relief will be provided by a dentist, who will remove the tooth or open a way into the tooth to allow gases and infection to escape.

If there is severe swelling and pain and you can't get to a dentist but can reach someone who can prescribe an antibiotic, this will help control the infection until a dentist can treat the tooth, which you should certainly arrange to have him do within a day or two.

As in most acute infections, the pain disappears after a few days. The gas breaks through the gum and bone and escapes. (You may see a "gum boil.") The pain is gone, but the infection remains.

When you examine a child's mouth after a toothache subsides, check the sides of all the teeth to see if there is a pimple along the gum near a decayed tooth. This is the pathway along which gas and pus escape. The child is constantly swallowing infectious matter, which lowers his resistance to other disease. Be sure that he sees a dentist as soon as possible.

against caries, trauma, and infection. When the nerves in the pulp begin to signal, it's important to pay attention, for infection can and often does spread from a tooth to the rest of the body. Understanding this is important in handling a toothache emergency.

Cementum

Just as the hard enamel laminates and protects the crown, or visible portion, of the tooth, the cementum — a thin, bonelike tissue — covers and protects the tooth root below the gums. It is not as hard as enamel and is less resistant to wear, as older people with receding gums too often find out. It forms fibers that, with other fibers formed by the bone, anchor the tooth to the bony socket and hold it in place.

The root makes up about two thirds of the total length of the tooth. The root is connected to the jawbone by special fibers that stretch like strips of elastic from the cementum-covering to the bone that lines the tooth socket. These are called periodontal fibers, or ligaments, and running through them are the blood vessels that supply nutrition to the cementum. When a dentist extracts a tooth, he is not breaking bone; he is just cutting the fiber that attaches the tooth to the bone. If teeth were actually part of the jaw, we couldn't remove a tooth without damage to the jawbone.

THE ENVIRONMENT OF THE TEETH

The environment the teeth find themselves in is an active one. The taste buds — those busy cells that tell us what we like and what we don't like — are here, and so are the salivary glands. Here are the lips, tongue, cheeks, and muscles of the jaw — the forces that are always pushing, pressing, moistening, and exerting environmental stress on the teeth.

Teeth are remarkable. They can detect a fine grit between them. Their ability to sense size resides in little pressure receptors in the periodontal fiber, not in the teeth themselves. It is interesting that teeth can't tell the difference between hot and cold. When a child bites into ice cream or drinks hot soup, the teeth may register pain. But it's the lips and tongue that have the temperature receptors.

Supporting Structures

The periodontal ligament anchoring the tooth's root to the jawbone is one of the surrounding structures of the tooth. We count the jawbone itself — also called the "alveolar bone" — as part of that structure; it's the bony portion of the upper and lower jaws that surrounds and supports the roots of the teeth and the gingiva, or gums. The health and integrity of these tissues are of vital importance to the tooth. A sound, cavity-free tooth is only as secure as the structures that hold and support it.

The gums are a good diagnostic tool in detecting vitamin deficiencies because they react early; the gums are also susceptible to other problems, particularly those caused by the buildup of hard, razor-sharp deposits of tartar (calculus) along the gum line. The gums move away from the bacteria that live on the tartar and, in so doing, move away from the tooth, allowing pockets to form, where food particles and bacteria are caught. Infection that begins here can damage the gums, beginning with inflammation and tiny tears in the surface tissue. The first sign of infection you may notice is bleeding of the gums when the teeth are brushed. The periodontal ligament is also susceptible to infection. Inflammation caused by toxins from the bacteria in the plaque around the neck of the tooth will loosen the periodontal attachment. Eventually, infection will reach the alveolar bone. Gum diseases are often found in older teen-agers and adults, but are sometimes diagnosed in children.

An interesting fact is that in a healthy mouth the response to hard use of all of these supporting structures — the gums, periodontal ligament, and alveolar bone — is their strengthening. For instance, the stress of chewing tough foods and the stress of vigorous brushing, shared evenly by the teeth, make the gums, ligaments, and bone stronger, and keep them in better tone. On the other hand, if an area of the mouth gets no use — because of missing teeth or because a malocclusion or a cavity discourages chewing in that area — then the tissues lose tone, the ligaments lose strength and elasticity, and the underlying alveolar bone may actually break down, decalcify, and be lost.

Old Wives' Tale

"When a youngster's gums bleed, just stay away from them. They will heal by themselves."

Not true. It's the food and bacteria that collect at the spot where the gums meet the teeth that are causing the trouble. Brush more effectively. In two or three days, the gums will usually toughen up and won't bleed so readily. They will continue to stay well unless you again fail to brush them properly.

Saliva

The salivary glands are located in the cheeks and in the floor of the mouth. When you are looking at your baby's mouth, familiarizing yourself with his "inside" as well as his "outside," locate and look at the openings of the parotid salivary glands in the cheeks so you won't be startled by them later and wonder what they are. They are small flaps of tissue, on the inside of both cheeks, that indicate the openings of the major salivary glands.

Saliva is a remarkable substance that performs several useful jobs in the mouth. A drop in the saliva output will trigger the sensation of thirst, reminding the body to take in more water and thus serving to regulate water balance. Saliva lubricates food, making chewing and swallowing easier. And it contains an enzyme that helps in the digestion of starches.

Saliva is very important to the well-being of the teeth. As air moves through the mouth, drying the teeth and the gum tissues, saliva remoistens them. Saliva also helps to wash the teeth free of food debris, but this doesn't mean you can give up your toothbrush. Nature needs all the help it can get.

One of the most remarkable properties of saliva is its buffering capacity — that is, its ability to neutralize acid. We know that acid is formed in the mouth when food debris is broken down by bacteria. This acid, held against the tooth in plaque, destroys the enamel and makes decay possible. The particular chemical make-up of saliva enables it to neutralize these acids.

There are some individuals who go through life without ever getting a cavity. Dental researchers are studying the saliva of these individuals in order to discover whether its composition holds the secret to their cavity-free state.

The Bacterial Population in Your Mouth

Also part of the teeth's environment are some eighty varieties of microorganisms — a fairly stable population in anybody's mouth. A recent important research discovery is that of these eighty or so different bacteria, only three or four are responsible for caries.* And, even more interesting, only certain kinds attack certain areas of the tooth. In other words, the bacteria that make holes on the biting surface of a tooth are different from those that make holes at the gum line or on the side. These three or four bacteria have two things in common that make them susceptible to destruction. They all need time to organize and sugar to survive. This information gives us the keys to defensive dentistry.

As we have seen, the tooth in its environment is pushed around by the dynamic forces of moving muscles, washed in a bath of saliva, affected by extremes of temperature as we feed ourselves hot dogs and ice cream, and is dried by the flow of air into and out of the lungs. The mouth is a busy crossroads of the body and important to our anatomy and to our psyche. We've had a close look at the tooth. Now let's visualize the tooth within the mouth, the mouth in the face, the face in the total person.

*Another important caries-research breakthrough of recent years shows that rats raised in a germ-free environment do not develop caries until rats with caries are introduced into the germ-free colony.

FOUR

A Complete Guide to Clean Teeth

There is a new approach to cleaning your teeth, and if someone has not demonstrated the technique for you, I'd like to take you through the basic steps so that you can teach it to your children. This method prevents cavities in children and gum disease in adults.

Remember the old advice, "Brush twice a day; see your dentist twice a year"? Good, but inadequate. The old method was intended for polishing teeth and removing food particles. The new way emphasizes plaque control.

WHAT IS PLAQUE?

During the time people were working to overcome resistance to the fluoridation of water supplies, researchers were busily attacking another menace to oral health — a transparent film that sticks tenaciously to the teeth and can hardly be seen. It's called plaque. It forms all the time, twenty-four hours a day. This sticky film is a mat on which bacteria breed. They quickly colonize in sheltered areas along the gum line, on surfaces next to other teeth, and in pits and fissures on molar surfaces.

Once established, the colony flourishes and expands, and other bacteria move in. Within a day or two, whole new organisms are thriving there, and as the early settlers (who are generally aerobic) use up the oxygen in the sticky layer, anaerobic bacteria begin to find a home in the new environment. Soon a complex little community is living on your teeth.

The unpleasant odor of bad breath usually comes from the gas created by the bacteria in the plaque. That's why strong mouthwashes work for only a short time. They disguise the smell but don't remove the plaque, with its gas-producing bacteria.

Plaque is the stuff you can scrape off your teeth with your fingernail. A milligram of plaque may contain as many as 200 to 500 million microorganisms. Yes, I know that the mouth always harbors bacteria, many of them harmless or even beneficial, but ordinary saliva contains fewer than 1 percent of the number of microorganisms just cited. And when all these acid-producing bugs are held against one area of a tooth — for hours and hours, perhaps for days — well, you can see why dentists recommend plaque control, even in an infant's mouth.

If plaque is left undisturbed, the bacteria multiply rapidly and form a gel-like matrix. It takes about twenty-four hours for dangerous amounts of sticky plaque to form on teeth. After this, it sometimes hardens and forms tartar, which you yourself can't scrape off with a toothbrush or a fingernail. The dentist or his dental hygienist must remove it with special tools.

Plaque and Decay

Think of plaque as a chemical factory in your mouth, continually producing strong acids that destroy teeth and gums.

A dark spot that appears on the surface of the tooth may be an early sign of decay. This is where the acids are dissolving the enamel surface of the tooth. Next, there's a hole; decay reaches the soft inner part of the tooth, and the destructive process speeds up. Finally, decay reaches the nerve center. If you haven't had a warning pain before, you'll have it now. Result: at best, a restorative filling; at worst, loss of the tooth.

Plaque and Periodontal Disease

These same bacteria, living in plaque, set the stage for periodontal or gum disease. Plaque creeps into the fold of tissue at the gum line, along the root of the tooth. As the bacteria die, they mineralize and become tartar. As plaque moves deeper into the gums, you'll notice inflamation, redness, puffiness. The condition may worsen until the supporting tissues pull away and the teeth literally fall out.

Of course, that's a horror story for grownups. Adults suffer more from periodontal disease than from decay. However, gum problems are not limited to adults; almost everybody experiences some degree of gingivitis (inflammation of the gums) at one time or another. Bleeding gums are a symptom of infection.

Researchers have demonstrated that if a normal human subject completely ceases practicing oral hygiene, gingivitis will result within two to three weeks. When oral hygiene and plaque-control methods are resumed, gingivitis clears up. It might be expected that if a person neglects oral hygiene indefinitely, loss of alveolar bone and loss of teeth will result. Experiments in this area have not been carried out because the end result, unlike gingivitis, is irreversible. A few days of vigorous brushing will clear up gingivitis in a child within a few days. You and the child will both have to suffer a bit first, however; the brushing initially makes the gums bleed more.

PLAQUE CONTROL

Now for the good news. Although your plaque factory works around the clock, plaque can be controlled. If the formation of plaque is interrupted once every twenty-four hours, it cannot hurt your teeth.

This is one of the key concepts of preventive dentistry, and it grew out of the research on plaque. If you spend a few minutes once a day brushing and flossing away plaque, you'll be taking the single most important step toward oral health. Only you can do it: you are the only one who can control the plaque in your mouth.

The old brushing technique called for up-and-down strokes with a hard-bristle brush, and for dental floss used occasionally to remove a recalcitrant food particle. The new way removes the plaque, and flossing is a must.

There are a number of acceptable toothbrushing methods that clean food debris from the teeth, but I want to suggest one — a kind of soft-scrub method that children can handle — that will remove plaque.

To instruct your child, try the soft-scrub stroke on his hand. Place the brush in the palm of his hand and move the bristles forward about one-half inch, without actually displacing the head of the brush. Flexing the bristles is all that is necessary. You'll produce a kind of jiggling or vibrating movement. Try it on your own hand and you'll see what I mean. Now lighten the pressure, speed up the movements, and there you have the soft-scrub stroke.

This is the way we teach. However, I don't insist on every point. If a child is more comfortable or more adept at brushing in a different direction — even in circles — it's fine with me.

A word of caution: excessive pressure can, indeed, wear away enamel. A soft brush and skill in its use are best.

Basic Brushing — Step by Step

1. Place the head of your toothbrush alongside your teeth, with the bristle tips angled against the gum line. Look at yourself in the mirror as you brush. I feel strongly that there should be a child-level mirror in every bathroom.
2. Move the brush back and forth with short strokes — about half a tooth wide. Use a gentle scrubbing motion, brushing one or two teeth at a time and then moving the brush on to the next couple of teeth.
3. Here is a way to brush the entire mouth systematically. Start with the last tooth and then move toward the front of the mouth on the outside. Still using the same short, back-and-forth strokes, brush the inside surfaces. Brush all four quarters of the mouth.
4. To brush the insides of the front teeth, tilt the brush vertically, angle the bristles toward your gums, and use short up-and-down strokes.
5. Now, keeping the brush flat, brush the chewing surfaces of your teeth. Don't forget the pits and grooves on molars — it's sometimes hard to clean these surfaces. You can even clean your tongue with your toothbrush — makes your mouth feel fresher.
6. Rinse vigorously. Smile.

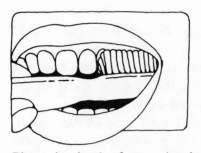

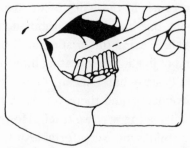

Place the head of your brush alongside your teeth, with the bristle tips angled against the gum line.

Brush the insides of front teeth with the "toe" (front part) of the brush.

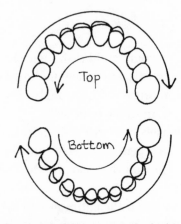

Brush the outsides and the insides of your upper and lower teeth.

HOW TO BRUSH YOUR TEETH

The Importance of Flossing

You may have used floss to dislodge bits of food caught between the teeth. Perhaps you never thought of it as a means for removing plaque — what I call shining the proximal sides of the teeth.

The places children most often miss are:

- the tongue side of all back molars,
- the cheek side of upper molars.

This is especially true of chubby children; there's not much room to get a brush between cheek and tooth.

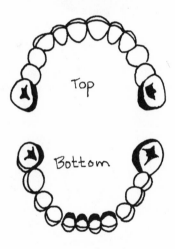

PLACES A CHILD MISSES MOST OFTEN

Even the best brush cannot completely remove plaque between the teeth and beneath the gum line. Flossing *does* remove plaque and debris from between the teeth and below the gum line — areas where decay often starts.

FLOSSING TECHNIQUE

One way to arrange the floss that may be easier for young children to manage is to take a piece of floss about twelve or fourteen inches long and knot the ends together so that the child has a circle to work with. The most important place for a youngster to floss is between the last two molars in each jaw. As he grows older and the natural spaces between his teeth grow smaller, he can become as adept as you in the method outlined below.

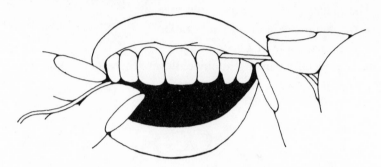

Use dental floss to clean the sides of your teeth. Floss goes under the gum line. It must clean tooth surfaces on both sides of every space.

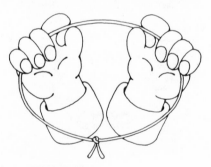

Holding floss tied in a circle.

FLOSSING YOUR TEETH

1. Break off about eighteen inches of floss and wind most of it around one of your middle fingers. The middle finger of the opposite hand can take up the used floss as you work on your teeth.
2. Holding the floss taut (there should be no slack), keep one inch free and, with a gentle, sawing motion, slide it between your teeth. Don't be rough.

3. When the floss reaches the gum line, curve it against a tooth, gently sliding it into the space between the gum and the tooth.
4. Holding the floss tightly against the tooth, scrape the floss up and down against the side of one tooth. Then curve it against the opposing tooth and again scrape up and down. This will break up the plaque and remove the bacteria.
5. Think of your mouth as having four sections; floss one section at a time. Once you establish a regular pattern, you can do it without thinking, and you won't miss any of your teeth.

Flossing is a skill that can be developed with a little practice. After you've flossed for a few days, you will find that it will take only a few minutes of your time. Flossing can be done anytime — while you're reading or watching television — but flossing at bedtime is best because it means a clean mouth throughout the nighttime hours. It will be twenty-four hours before plaque again reaches a critical plateau.

Other Cleaning Aids

Brushing and flossing are the basic tools of plaque control. They are the easiest, best, least expensive ways to remove plaque from the teeth and gums.

THE RIGHT TOOTHBRUSH

Adopt a new attitude toward your old friend the toothbrush. It's not just something to make your teeth attractive, it's a weapon for attacking plaque. The right brush for the method of brushing described on page 83 has a straight handle, soft bristles, a flat brushing surface, at least three rows of bristles, a small head.

A soft nylon brush with double-rounded, small bristles is good. The tufts of the bristles should all be the same length. The head of the brush should be small enough so that children can reach all the teeth in their mouth, at the gum line as well as the grooved molar surfaces.

Everybody should (need I say it?) use only his or her own toothbrush and replace it promptly when it begins to wear out. Store it in a place where it will dry quickly and won't touch other brushes. Have two toothbrushes on hand and use them alternately, and maybe even one more toothbrush in reserve in case the bristles of your old brush begin to look frayed, limp, and loose.

It takes a day for a nylon toothbrush to dry out. If a child is using the same brush every day, it gets soft — too soft to do an adequate job.

The same points apply to the brushing head of an electric toothbrush. A powered brush, used properly, can be effective, and can be especially helpful for a handicapped child. But if a person is going to brush carelessly with a regular toothbrush, he'll do the same with an electric device.

Electric toothbrushes are more efficient than manual toothbrushes. However, they have major problems. Like other "labor-saving" electric devices stored in odd corners of the bathroom and kitchen, electric toothbrushes get to be too much trouble to get out, assemble, and use every day. Then, too, parents buy electric toothbrushes in the hope that they will encourage children to brush. The novelty works only for a while — as with any new toy.

I would buy an electric brush only for the child who has already developed the habit of cleaning his teeth every day. Otherwise, it will soon be available for cleaning the algae off the sides of fish tanks or for shining shoes.

MOUTHWASHES

Mouthwashes temporarily freshen breath and sweeten the mouth, but do not remove plaque and cannot prevent dental disease. In fact, their use may mask a condition that needs professional attention. The fluoride mouthwashes do bring fluoride in contact with the teeth. They should be used at the end of cleaning.

WATER IRRIGATING DEVICES

Oral irrigating devices that shoot small jets of water between and around teeth will flush out loose debris and can be especially helpful to children wearing braces, teen-agers with wisdom teeth, and older people with bridgework. They feel good. They don't, however, remove plaque; they're not a substitute for brushing. Plaque is too tenacious.

INTERDENTAL DEVICES

Besides dental floss, other interdental devices are available. They include rubber-tipped probes, toothpicklike instruments, and wooden, plastic, and quill devices. I wouldn't give these to a child. They are of questionable value in removing plaque from youngsters' teeth, and can scratch and injure gum tissue.

While we are taking a look at misconceptions about plaque removal, let me list some other things that have been shown *not* to be effective substitutes for brushing and flossing:

- eating crisp food,
- rinsing the mouth with water,
- chewing gum.

Old Wives' Tale

"Chewing gum helps clean the teeth and prevent decay."
Now I wonder what chewing gum manufacturer started this one? No, chewing gum does not clean teeth — only brushing and flossing will clean teeth. And what's more to the point, a stick of ordinary gum contains approximately half a teaspoon of sugar — and sugar, especially between meals, can only be bad news for teeth.

I am *not* against chewing gum. Chewing is good exercise for the jaw, and it relieves tension. Just remember that sugarless gums are available.

WHAT DENTIFRICE IS BEST?

Any fluoride-containing dentifrice that is recognized by the American Dental Association as being effective in reducing tooth decay is recommended. Dentifrices have a number of advantages:

- They are excellent vehicles for bringing fluoride in contact with the tooth surface. The more times and the more ways fluoride is brought in contact with a tooth, the stronger that tooth will be and the more resistant to decay.

• Dentifrices contain a detergent material that helps the brush sweep away some of the debris found on teeth.

• Dentifrices have a pleasant taste and leave your mouth feeling refreshed after you've brushed.

You might ask, "If the water supply is fluoridated, is it really that beneficial to use a fluoride dentifrice?" Yes — most definitely. The uptake of fluoride is a surface phenomenon. New research shows that topical fluoride provides a benefit in addition to that which comes from fluoride in your drinking water.

DISCLOSING TABLETS

How can you tell when your child's teeth are really clean? You can locate the plaque on teeth by using disclosing tablets or liquids that temporarily color the plaque red. These are made from harmless vegetable dyes. The color will disappear gradually but completely. Be sure to explain the experiment to a child carefully beforehand; he'll be interested in the process. The tablets are inexpensive and can be purchased at any drugstore, or perhaps your dentist will give you some. I find disclosing tablets to be a good teaching device. My children use them at least once a week. A small piece of one tablet is adequate for most children.

Check yourself out, along with your children. Chew a tablet for thirty seconds without swallowing. Now rinse your mouth out with water. Swish the liquid all around the teeth, then spit. Examine your teeth in a good source of light so that you can see their inner and outer surfaces. Study the pattern of plaque accumulation in your mouth. Every mouth is different. There is considerable individual variation in the amount of plaque formed and in its distribution in different parts of the mouth.

You'll probably see that the areas with the darkest stains are between the teeth, along the gum line, on any roughened surface or crack, and on any area that is protected from lip, tongue, and cheek action by the tooth's shape or position. These will probably always be the places you should concentrate your cleaning efforts on. (See page 85 for the places children most often miss.)

Use a disclosing tablet periodically to see how well you are cleaning your teeth. It's a good way to check yourself.

TIPPING THE SCALE TOWARD NO DECAY

There is an interesting clinical phenomenon that I see as a dentist. Of two children in the same family, one may have a history of decay and the other may reach the age of twelve or fourteen without having had a single cavity. People point to these two children and say, "They live in the same house, are given the same foods, have the same things happening to them. Why the difference? Does one have something in his genetic inheritance that blessed him with decay-resistant teeth?"

In my mind there is very little in heredity that bears on dental decay. The real difference between these two children is their habits. One may brush his teeth aggressively; the other, halfheartedly. One may like crisp foods; the other may prefer soft foods. Differences like these may seem very slight, but they add up. I call the sum, and the components, of these differences the etiologic pile.

What I mean by this is that there is a host of factors that can cause dental breakdown, and it's not until the pile of accumulated factors reaches a certain height that the scale for one individual is tipped toward decay.

Teeth are marvelous natural things and have a great resistance to decay. The best way to prevent decay is to understand all the factors that can tip the scales the wrong way, and then work toward lifting those factors you have control over off the negative side of the scale, so that the scale is balanced on the side of prevention — not tipped toward decay.

Now, what is this etiologic pile composed of — what are some of the factors stacked up here that can tip the scale toward caries? To list them, you first have to understand the caries process.

The simplest way is to think of a tooth as a child's wooden block.

In your mind, picture that block with a lump of clay stuck to it. Suspended in the clay are lots of tiny beads. The clay is the plaque, which sticks to the block and holds the bacteria against the block's surface. The tiny beads are the bacteria that continue to live and thrive there.

Bacteria

Ideally, there would be a vaccine against those particular organisms that cause dental caries. Such a vaccine is not here yet, and it's doubtful that one will be developed.

Another futuristic solution would be a strain of bacteria you could drop into your mouth that would crowd out the caries-producing bacteria. That's not on the books yet, either.

Still another suggestion, one that has been tried with laboratory animals for a long time, is the use of penicillin or antibiotics to cut down a broad range of flora in the mouth. In these experiments, no matter what diet the lab animals are fed — even tons of sugar and soft carbohydrates — they don't get dental caries. But the problem in giving antibiotics to *people* is that people eventually build up antibiotic-resistant bacteria in their mouths, and sooner or later the effect is nil and decay comes along.

Getting rid of the bacteria is not the answer for the present, but it is the area where most dental research is going on. The ideal agent will probably turn out to be something we can add to our water supply, like fluoride, that will kill the bacteria in people's mouths that are caries-producing and leave the other ones alone. However, for now we must concentrate on ridding the teeth of the substance produced by the bacteria.

Plaque

The ever-constant formation of plaque is the next factor in our etiologic pile. Plaque contains a sticky substance called "dextran." It is secreted by the bacteria. Scientists are working on an enzyme called "dextranase," which will break up plaque. If they could introduce it into a breakfast cereal, it would cause plaque on the tooth's surface to become loose, and would keep more plaque from forming. Without a home, bacteria are out in the cold; there's no way for them to hold on to the tooth. Therefore, there's no acid and no holes.

It's important to understand that bacteria eat sugar, and that the acid that is the waste product of the bacteria is what makes the first tiny hole in the enamel. The bacteria, ingesting the sugar, produce dextran (that's the sticky "clay" in our example), which provides a home for more bacteria, which, in turn, produce more dextran, more plaque and more acid, the substance that breaks down the tooth. Not only does sugar feed the bacteria and keep them turning out acid, but it also gives them the material to make dextran.

THE TOOTH'S SURFACE

The surface of the tooth is naturally hard, and is impermeable to the penetration of acid unless the acid is there for an appreciable period of time. A tooth's surface is usually bathed with saliva, which, besides keeping the tooth moist, contains substances whose buffering effect neutralizes acids. One way to make the tooth's surface stronger is to incorporate fluoride into it. This, too, will help to keep down the etiologic pile and avoid decay.

Enamel is a crystal structure composed of several elements. One of its molecules (the hydroxyl, or OH, molecule) can be replaced with a molecule of a harder mineral — fluoride — if it is present when the tooth is forming. If this substitution takes place, the crystal matrix of the tooth is all the more resistant to acid.

There are a number of ways to get fluoride into the crystal. You can do it topically — in an application in the dentist's office; through a fluoride mouthwash; through use of a dentifrice that contains fluoride; through the topical effect of fluoridated water as it passes through the mouth — or systemically, by getting fluoride into the body's system in the early years as the teeth are forming (more exactly, the years from birth to age five). See Chapter 6 for a complete discussion of fluoride.

Sealants

One method of keeping plaque and acid off the teeth is to use sealants. A sealant is a coat of plastic material applied to the biting

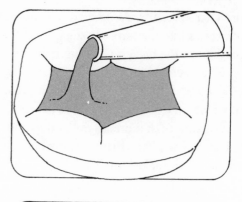

Sealant flowing
into crevice to
seal out decay

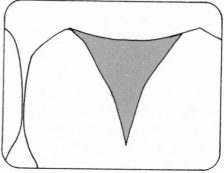

Crevice filled
with sealant

surface of the tooth so that the plaque and the bacteria have a layer
of plastic between them. Then the bacteria can make all the acid they
want; it won't penetrate the sealant. Sealants for tooth surfaces are
already past the experimental stage and are in use, especially for the
biting surfaces of molars. Sealants for the entire tooth are under
study.

Contouring Teeth

Another technique that dentists have known for a long time but
practice infrequently is reshaping the occlusal biting surfaces of the
molars, grinding away the tiny nooks and crannies that tend to cause
food particles and bacteria to get trapped and stick to the teeth. The
dentist makes the surface saucerlike instead of like little valleys and
craters. He sculpts a smoother surface, which discourages food from
accumulating, thus cutting down on the formation of plaque. Con-

touring the teeth is not bad so long as the dentist stays within the enamel area of the tooth. It's actually just rushing nature a little bit — most people wear these deep grooves down over the years anyway.

YOUR CHILD'S ETIOLOGIC PILE

Even if your child doesn't take all the steps, if she does enough *for her as an individual,* she'll balance her scale on the side of *no decay.* And that's whether she eats candy or doesn't eat candy, or brushes twice a day or three times.

For a child up to the age of eight or so, the best insurance is still supervised brushing — what I call the buddy system. If a child doesn't wash her face and hands, she can't get away with it very long — the evidence is pretty hard to conceal. But if she forgets to brush her teeth, very likely she can fake it for a long time. A toothbrushing buddy can be an older brother or sister or a parent. It adds to the control and accuracy of her cleaning program — and down goes the etiologic pile to another level.

You can tip your child's scale toward no decay with these four basic tips.

1. Effective toothbrushing supervised by a parent or by a tooth-brushing buddy two times a day — and at the right times of the day. By right times, I mean after breakfast before going to school, and at night after the last time the child eats.
2. Fluoride in the water supply, topical fluoride applied at the dentist's office approximately every six months, and the use at home of a fluoride dentifrice and mouthwash.
3. An understanding that between-meal snacks and sugary foods will feed the bacteria that produce the acid that makes the holes in teeth.
4. Cutting down on the *number* of sugar challenges a tooth faces in a day. One orgy of sweets, so long as it's followed by brushing, is going to do the teeth no harm.

FIVE

Diet Decisions

Nutrition is a neglected science. The information just doesn't get to the average person. If it does, it is so obscured by advertising, and so negated by what we actually see and hear, that even when we know better, we don't do better. Your child's schoolroom may have bright posters on the wall, illustrating the four basic food groups with bright colors and attractive graphics, but the school lunchroom and the snack machines convey a different message.

Although some dentists include nutrition counseling in their preventive program, many prefer to concentrate on bringing about behavioral changes in the oral hygiene habits of their patients rather than on trying to alter their dietary patterns. I suppose they feel that to attempt to change two areas of behavior simultaneously may be too difficult and discouraging.

NUTRITION AND TEETH

As for the connection between nutrition and teeth, it's difficult, even among experts, to draw specific conclusions. Experiments with hamsters and other laboratory animals are sometimes inconclusive, and it's hard to experiment with people. Even if we had enough control populations on whom to conduct studies, each of the people in these groups would still have different patterns of mineralization, a different heritage in tooth structure, a different chewing pattern, different saliva, different metabolism. Current studies seem to indicate that, though diet is important to the whole system, the most important effect of food on the teeth is local — that is, while food is in actual contact with the teeth.

Dental caries is a multifactorial disease. There is not *just one thing* that causes it. It takes a whole pile of factors to tip your child's situation toward cavities. We think that what the child eats is one of the heaviest items on the scale, and one of the easiest to manage a change in — if you try. What it really takes is a high degree of determination and self-discipline.

YOU ARE WHAT YOU EAT, BUT . . .

I must tell you now that you can eat well and wisely and still have decay. The strongest, best-formed teeth decay just as rapidly as the poorest in an environment that invites caries — that is, in a mouth where:

- too many soft, high-carbohydrate, sugar-filled foods linger too long,
- there is an unfavorable oral bacteria count due to poor hygiene,
- teeth are unprotected by fluoride,
- plaque formation is not being controlled on a daily basis,
- teeth are brushed, but at the wrong times, or a poor job is being done, with no one checking up.

You see, good nutrition contributes to good health, but diet alone is no insurance in our plan to have children with strong, disease-free teeth.

WHAT AND WHEN TO EAT

What to eat and when and how much and how often are all factors you can control. Even if you, as a parent, can't run an absolutely tight ship (it gets progressively harder as children get older and have access to foods away from home), you can make the most intelligent choices and decisions you know how to about what to eat and when

Diet Analysis: A Profile of Your Child's Day

If you can answer the following questions about your child's eating habits through the day, you should have a picture that will tell you a lot about the quality, quantity, and physical consistency of the food your child eats, as well as about the frequency of food intake.

- What does your child like to eat?
- What does your child eat between meals?
- What did your child have for breakfast this morning?
- What do other people (Grandma, the school, the babysitter) feed your child?
- What do you give your child for a snack?
- Do you give your child food before he goes to bed?
- If your child forages for his own snacks after school and at other times, what does he choose?
- Does your child buy food for himself with his allowance or lunch money?
- When does your child brush? Before or after breakfast? An hour after the evening meal?
- Are foods — especially dessert foods — used as rewards or special treats at your house?
- Do you adhere to the same nutrition rules you make for your child?

to eat it, and explain these decisions to your family. Diet is the do-it-yourself side of preventive dentistry.

You need information about the effect of food on teeth, and this means more than nutrition alone. Food has much of its effect while it is in the mouth, and this effect has to do with the food's content, consistency, and frequency in the diet. Your child's dental health can be improved more by changing not what he eats but when he eats it.

It would be great to stop the production and distribution of sugar, but we can't do that. Understanding that it's the number of times during the day that sugar comes in contact with teeth, being aware of the "stickies" — insidious foods that hold sugar to the tooth's surface — and being able to substitute non-sugar-containing snacks for them in your youngster's diet will make up for the fact that sugar is something we have to live with.

Foods containing sugar trigger acid formation almost immediately. Enamel-destroying acid is active for at least twenty minutes before it is totally buffered or dispersed by the flow of saliva; so for at least that long, your teeth are bathed in acid. If you restrict the number of times you eat to three meals a day, it means that your teeth are subjected to acid for about sixty minutes every day. Just think how that time increases if you have several snacks or soft drinks between meals and another snack at bedtime! It could be that your teeth are exposed to an acid bath for several hours each day. And if the snacks you choose are sweet or sticky or both, you're headed for disaster.

Old Wives' Tale

"Children need sugar for energy!"

Children need energy, but there are better places to find it than in refined sucrose, with its empty calories. Other foods provide plenty of energy, and bring with them the bonus of other essential nutrients.

If your child has an extraordinarily stressful dilemma to face in getting to school — such as swimming a channel against an incoming tide, or fighting off the wild animals that roam between your house and the school door — there may be some reason for a sugar-loaded breakfast, which does indeed become a potential source of quick energy. If it's needed. If it's not, this carbohydrate high is going to be followed by a let-down.

Perhaps our primordial ancestors' sweet tooth led them to the fruits and berries that were their only source of vitamin C. But today our sweet tooth leads each of us to consume nearly 100 pounds of sugar every year. That's a spoonful every few minutes!

Old Wives' Tale

"Raw sugar is less harmful to your teeth than white, refined sugar."

Here are the scientific facts. Raw sugar, after extraction from the plant, contains 98 percent sucrose along with 2 percent water, invert sugar, and natural impurities. After refining, white sugar contains 99.9 percent sucrose. We're talking about a difference of less than 2 percent in sucrose content. The bacteria on your teeth will never notice the difference.

All sugar feeds the microorganisms on your teeth. The sugar in an orange, in the sugar bowl, in a raisin — it's all the same to them.

SNACKS: THE GOOD GUYS AND THE BAD GUYS

Here's a list of the sticky, easily fermentable foods that are most responsible for tooth decay. If your children eat them, impress on them the importance of rushing to brush.

The Sugar Stickies

Chocolate milk, condensed milk, cocoa, all kinds of soda, sweet sauces, sweetened fruit-flavored drinks (these are no substitute for fruit juice), white bread, pastries, cakes, cookies, macaroni, spaghetti, jams and jellies, ice cream, dried fruits, candy (especially sticky or hard, long-lasting candies), marshmallows, chewing gum, processed or presweetened cereals, raisins.

Start very early, with a rule a child can understand: if it's sweet and sticky, it's bad for your teeth. If you *must* eat it, brush immediately afterward. *It's what stays in the mouth that starts decay!*

If you can't brush but still feel you must eat it, then eat it at mealtime and eat a piece of fruit or part of your green salad afterward.

If you are in the middle of Grand Central Station and you cannot brush but still feel you must eat it, then take a mouthful of water afterward, swish, and swallow. This will wash away some of the sugar that would otherwise stay on your teeth.

I realize that food is more than just something to eat. Often it satisfies an emotional need, too. If your children must have sweets — and remember, this is largely a matter of conditioning, not a real physical need — try to serve sweets under controlled conditions: after dinner, just before everybody cleans his or her teeth, or before the conclusion of a meal that then ends with a crisp salad or an apple or a pear. Eliminate sugar-filled snacks that constitute a constant attack on teeth through the day. It takes very little sugar to feed those bacteria living in plaque.

Here are some snack ideas that will stave off starvation but won't turn on the acid. A handy supply of these in the kitchen may keep teen-agers from the junk foods their friends are subsisting on.

Nutritious Snacks

Hard-boiled or deviled eggs
Fresh fruits
Olives, pickles, sauerkraut
Cheese cubes or slices
Raw, fresh vegetables, ready to eat: bell-pepper strips, celery and
  carrot sticks, cherry tomatoes, cabbage and lettuce wedges, sliced
  cucumbers, cauliflower pieces, radishes
Fresh coconut chunks
Popcorn
Fresh fruit juices (to combat fruit-flavored drinks and soda, which are
  higher in sugar)
Orange-juice ices (orange juice, frozen in ice-cube trays)
Plain yogurt
Soups (a good snack, any time of day, cold or hot)
Cheese-stuffed celery
Nuts
Snacks of mixed nuts, pretzel sticks, potato chips, corn chips (nutri-
  tious but sticky — be prepared to brush after these foods)
Finger sandwiches made with whole-grain breads

I'm suggesting not so much a change in diet as that certain foods — such as dried fruits, presweetened cereals, jams, honey, ice cream, chocolate milk, foods found to be both sweet and long-staying in the mouth — be eaten at mealtime, and avoided as snacks.

THE BREAKFAST HABIT

Many children with serious decay eat a high-carbohydrate breakfast. I recommend a high-protein breakfast — one containing, for example, fortified milk, two eggs, and cottage cheese or cheese toast made with whole-grain bread. Furthermore, what the child eats for breakfast seems to be easier to alter than some other eating patterns in the child's life. Most important, once breakfast is right, there is rarely a serious problem of widespread decay occurring again.

Other foods contain the same energy potential as sugar; they just take a few more minutes to be digested and absorbed by the tissues. And other foods contain things that sugar doesn't: proteins, vitamins, fats, and minerals, all essential for health and growth. A super-sweet breakfast not only feeds those cavity-causing bacteria, it also gives your child a sugar "high," which he doesn't need and which keeps him from getting food that will provide a steady, natural level of energy until lunchtime.

Breakfast doesn't have to be boring. There is a conventional aspect to breakfast that some people find repetitious, but you don't have to stick to the clichés. There's no reason why you can't start the day with a bowl of hot soup or a toasted peanut butter sandwich — or, if you're a teen-ager, with a hamburger.

Here's a list of breakfast suggestions, including some unconventional choices that will add variety to breakfast without sacrificing nutrition.

Novel Breakfast Suggestions

Grilled-cheese sandwiches
Cornmeal muffins
Brown rice — cooked with milk, with or without raisins
Cooked whole-grain cereals — served with butter or with fruit instead of sugar

Hamburgers or hot dogs

Corned-beef hash

Whole-wheat bread or toast — with toppings of bacon bits, banana slices, cheese, peanut butter

Fish fillets (quick and simple to prepare)

Eggs — cooked any way (An egg contains just about every nutritional element the body needs except vitamin C. Eggs are real protein bombs — and don't load you down with calories.)

Whole-wheat pancakes

Potato pancakes

Corn fritters

Fresh fruit and cheese cubes (quick and easy)

Cottage cheese

Fresh-fruit shakes — made with milk

It's hard for some people (parents as well as children) not to eat cereals at breakfast time and not to use sugar, syrup, or jelly on their food. At least be sure that your child brushes at the best time — after breakfast, before going to school. Too many children brush their teeth in the morning when they first get up. That's the *worst* time!

My children enjoy presweetened cereals. I feel that it would be unrealistic to ban them in my house. A bowl of presweetened cereal with milk does contain some nutritional elements. I have no objection to my children having the combination for breakfast. Remem-

---

Old Wives' Tale

"Why should my children have cavities? I give them plenty of milk to drink."

No amount of milk will prevent tooth decay. It's true that milk is the best source of calcium, a mineral necessary to the healthy growth of teeth and bones, and children need milk daily as long as they are growing. Once the crowns of the teeth are fully formed, calcium intake ceases to have much effect. Remember, in a bad environment, the strongest teeth can deteriorate as rapidly as susceptible teeth.

ber, though, the rule in my house is that the children must *always* brush after breakfast.

Presweetened cereals are forbidden as between-meal snacks. Dry, they are as tooth-threatening as large lollipops. Look carefully at the advertising on TV — cereal manufacturers would never dare to advertise their presweetened products as between-meal snacks. The American Dental Association would jump all over them.

Good Choices and Bad Choices

If we as parents can make intelligent food choices, we will show our children how to do the same. And we'd better start now, for while custom and family eating patterns used to introduce children to nutrition, television is today's prompter. Food companies are the largest single group of advertisers on television. Many of the products they feature are the same refined, high-carbohydrate, sugar-saturated foods and soft drinks that abound in the supermarkets.

Early enchantment with appealing brand names and attractive, repeated commercials begins with toddlers and carries right into the teen years, so teen-agers, who need good nutrition more than anybody else except pregnant women and growing infants, are snacking their way through a period of rapid growth, developmental stress, and caries susceptibility. Bad choices lead to bad patterns, and the bad choices are getting easier and easier to make.

A new TV regulation in the Netherlands is trying to get across a little subliminal message. All candy advertisements must display a picture of a toothbrush and toothpaste on the screen. The concept of brushing may eventually become firmly associated with the concept of sweets.

We can do something similar through repetition: "If you choose sugar foods for a snack, you'll have to stop what you're doing and go and brush your teeth." My own children often find it's not worth it, and reach for a carrot instead of a cookie.

SIX

The Fluoride Story

Fluoridation, the most effective and economical method of strengthening the tooth against decay, is one of the greatest achievements in the history of public health protection. It ranks right along with vaccination, pasteurization, and chlorination — all public health measures that were controversial in their time.

A community that has decided to drink fluoridated water has, in effect, decided to reduce dental disease in its children by 50 to 75 percent. Because fluoridation saves money as well as teeth, the cost of dental care in that community is reduced. Chicago, one of the first major cities to fluoridate its water (1956), saved more than $20 million in dental bills in the first fifteen years of fluoridation, when tooth decay dropped by 50 percent among its school population.

What is fluoride? What does it do? How is it used? How safe is it? Does it do adults any good?

These are some of the questions people ask about fluoride. I am particularly interested in answering them, because one of the formative experiences of my life occurred when, as a young dental student, I worked on the historic Kingston-Newburgh experiment. The story of fluoride is an intriguing tale, one of the best real detective stories. In 1901 a dentist who had just graduated and started his practice in Colorado Springs began puzzling over the fact that his young patients had brown stains and mottling on their teeth that he could not remove. "It's the water," local residents said. That was only a kind of folk wisdom, because today's sophisticated methods of chemical analysis had not been developed. There were lots of theories about the stain but no scientific explanation.

By communicating with dentists in other areas and working with the U.S. Public Health Service, the young dentist eventually found that water was, indeed, the cause of the unsightly brown stain. The water in Colorado Springs — principally supplied from melted snow pouring down the mineral-bearing deposits on the slopes of Pikes Peak — contained a high count of dissolved fluorides.

As dentists began to focus on the cause of mottling — "Colorado Brown Stain," as the condition was sometimes called (*dental fluorosis* is the technical term) — they made another amazing discovery: children who had teeth marred by fluorosis also had teeth that were remarkably resistant to decay. Could something that made teeth look bad also be good for them?

As more studies were performed, it was discovered that too much fluoride in water caused mottling, but just enough brought enormous benefits.

"Just enough" turned out to be one part fluoride to one million parts water (1 ppm). This was established in rigorous tests, such as the one in which I took part in Newburgh, a community in New York State that decided to fluoridate its water (to 1.1 ppm), while Kingston, a neighboring city with fluoride-deficient water (0.1 ppm), served as a control.

There was a constant downward trend in caries in Newburgh's children, with the younger children showing the greatest benefits.

Newburgh (fluoridated)	**Kingston** (nonfluoridated)
41% of the 5- and 6-year-olds had no cavities.	17% of the 5- and 6-year-olds had no cavities.
Mean annual cost for dental treatment at age 5 was $13.86.	Mean annual cost for dental treatment at age 5 was $33.73.
Mean annual cost for dental treatment at age 6 was $16.93.	Mean annual cost for dental treatment at age 6 was $40.78.

Very thorough medical comparisons were made — growth rates, tonsillectomy rates, skeletal maturation, bone density — every test that could be thought of. The conclusion of long-term pediatric studies was that there was no indication of *any* effects, good or bad, from the use of fluoridated water — except for the reduction in cavities.

Let's look at another town's experience. Antigo, Wisconsin, after eleven years of fluoridating its water supply, reversed its decision and stopped. Within six years, the caries rate in kindergartners had gone up 112 percent. The town changed its mind and went back to fluoridated water.

A fluoridated water supply is extremely safe. How safe is extremely safe? There is nothing anywhere — in scientific literature, in test reports, in statistics, in the history of people who drank naturally fluoridated water long before some communities decided to add fluoride to their water supplies — to indicate or suggest that fluoride ever had a bad effect on anybody.

A lot of questions have been raised by antifluoride groups, but by and large, not one of them has had anything interesting or relevant to say. When analyzed, their arguments have much to do with attitudes that are antigovernmental and antiscientific, but very little to do with whether fluoridation works as a protection against dental disease.

I think the main reason why every community in the United States doesn't have a fluoridated water supply is simply that local authorities don't want to spend the money. They have decided it isn't worth it. They don't know that it helps everybody — adults, teen-agers, and, most of all, the children in the community.

WHAT ARE FLUORIDES?

Fluorides are a large group of chemical compounds formed from *fluorine* combining with other elements. Fluorine is a volatile reactive chemical element that is never found by itself in nature. Fluorides are found everywhere — in soil, in the air, in plant and animal life, in foods, and dissolved in water.

Minerals are unevenly distributed in the soil of the world, so it follows that the water and plants in one region may contain a high fluoride count, while those of another contain a low count. What we eat and drink will not supply these diet elements in a steady, balanced way, so we sometimes add them to our diets in the proper amounts.

We call fluoride an additive, but it is not really that. We are supplementing the fluoride in — not introducing it to — the water supply, adjusting the proportions to achieve the optimum balance that will enhance the strength of teeth.

Why the water supply? For one thing, it's the principal natural source of fluorides. As a public health measure, fluoridating water is the one way to reach the most people. We have other ways of adding fluoride to the diet, but they would require every parent and every child to be responsible for the additional fluoride every day. Such a system would never fit into the commitment to prevention — for today and for future generations.

HOW DOES FLUORIDE WORK?

The hardest substances in the body are bones and teeth. When the teeth are forming, the minerals needed are brought to the jaw and deposited in the tooth buds by the bloodstream. When one of these minerals, fluoride, is in adequate supply, it gets incorporated into the enamel of the tooth, and the resulting mineral structure is stronger than it would be without the fluoride. As a result, the enamel will be more resistant to attack by the acids that form in the mouth and set the stage for decay.

It's important, then, to get fluoride to the teeth when they are mineralizing. That means from birth, when the primary teeth are forming, right through the development of the adult molars and, in the case of wisdom teeth, even later. A child who has had fluoridated water to drink from infancy through the age of twelve or thirteen has teeth that are stronger than they would otherwise be. He can expect to have half the number of cavities — or even fewer — than he would have had. This is a lifetime advantage. The teeth are permanently stronger because fluoride has gone into their structure.

Popular Misconceptions About Fluoridation

1. Misconception: That Fluoride Causes Cancer

   Fact: Epidemiologic studies comparing death rates from cancer show no significant differences between fluoridated and non-fluoridated communities.

2. Misconception: That Fluoride Causes Kidney Dysfunction

   Fact: Studies show no differences in kidney function rates among residents of cities with varying amounts of fluoride in their drinking water.

3. Misconception: That Fluoride Causes Heart Disease

   Fact: Long-term fluoridation does not adversely affect cardiovascular disease mortality rates.

4. Misconception: That Fluoride Causes Allergies

   Fact: The fluoride levels used in water supplies are too low to cause allergic reactions.

5. Misconception: That Fluoride Causes Blood Anomalies

   Fact: Laboratory tests comparing populations consuming fluoridated and nonfluoridated water reveal no significant differences in the incidence of blood anomalies.

6. Misconception: That Fluoridation Equipment Is Not Safe

   Fact: The development and use of reliable continuous fluoride analyzers in conjunction with modern fluoride-feed systems assure safe communal water supplies.

Grownups may wonder what, if any, advantage fluoridated water has for them. It's true that adulthood is too late to build fluoride into the crystal matrix of the teeth, since adults' teeth are already formed, but fluoridated water serves the whole family by providing a *surface* benefit. This surface action is all you can expect, once the teeth are formed. Still, it's part of the total shield we're trying to erect against decay.

GETTING FLUORIDE INTO THE TOOTH

Fluoride taken internally is systemic — it will be incorporated into the system as building blocks. There are several ways of getting fluoride into the teeth systemically. When the drinking water in your community is fluoridated, the effect is both systemic and local, and it benefits everybody. Where this is not possible — in rural areas, for example — there can be fluoridation of school drinking water. For children who live in areas with nonfluoridated water, fluoride supplements are available as liquid solutions, in tablet form, and in preparations that combine fluoride with vitamins.

If you are going to give your child a fluoride supplement at home, it's important for both you and your child to understand how it should be administered and how often. Your dentist will determine the proper dosage, prescribe the appropriate type of supplement, and teach you how to use it. For instance, we think now that when giving a small child a liquid fluoride solution (one that can be dispensed with a medicine dropper or drip bottle), best results are achieved by placing the solution right on the tongue or inside the cheek. Parents used to be instructed to add it to water, formula, or juice, but the liquids dilute it, and reduce its effectiveness in conferring topical benefits.

Your dentist will consider your child's age when prescribing a fluoride supplement. Experts now question the value of prescribing fluoride supplements to childen younger than six months.

When children become old enough to manage chewable tablets, they can switch from the infant preparations. Best results from these are obtained if they are used after brushing and flossing, when the mouth is clean; they should be chewed well and swished around in the mouth before swallowing. Just remember to treat fluoride supplements like medicine. Store them out of reach of children and use as directed. Since there is such wide variation in levels of naturally occurring fluoride, it is best to have a physician or dentist write the prescription for fluoride supplementation for your child.

Making Fluoride Work Better for You

1. Fluoride goes into a clean tooth more easily than into a dirty tooth. Fluoride dentifrices and fluoride mouthwashes work better on clean teeth, and rinsing with fluoridated water after the teeth have been cleaned has a local effect.
2. Topical applications of fluoride are highly effective for children. The effect is additive: the more times fluoride is brought in contact with the teeth, the more protection the child gets.

It may be that even in an area with fluoridated water some infants are not getting the benefits of the mineral. If your child is very young, still an infant, take a look at your daily routine and ask yourself if he or she is actually drinking water. Is the bottle full of prepared formula or bottled juices instead? If so, make some of his or her food with tap water each day.

Does More Fluoride Mean More Protection?

There's another way to get fluoride into the tooth. In a topical solution — gel, paste, or liquid — it can be wiped or painted or swished around the surface of the tooth.

When you and your child are in the dentist's office for a periodic checkup and prophylaxis (cleaning), the dentist may suggest a series of topical fluoride treatments for the child.

The protective benefits of topical fluoride treatments are the key to the dental health of children living in communities with nonfluoridated water. But they are also important to children who do drink fluoridated water. For the average child, they add a little more weight on his side of the scale — that is, the chances that he'll have a cavity in the months after treatment drop a few more points. For the child suffering from serious, extensive caries, topical treatments can help slow up a runaway situation.

Sometimes I'm faced with such a severe case of caries that pull out all stops and try everything — reviewing cleaning techniques, checking the diet, and recommending a daily rinse with a fluoride solution. Home use of topical fluorides — the same kind I use in my office — may be prescribed until things start looking better.

Topical Fluoride Treatments

After your child's teeth have been cleaned and carefully dried, the dentist will apply fluoride. Most preparations have a pleasant taste, and the treatment lasts only a few minutes.

One method is to fill a tray, molded to fit the teeth, with a solution or gel and place it over the teeth for a few minutes. Another way is to apply the fluoride solution with cotton applicators and carry it between the teeth with dental floss. Dentists are studying still other methods of applying topical fluoride to teeth, including the use of fluoride-containing chewing gum and fluoridated dental floss.

Fluoride in Dentifrices

Even if your water supply is fluoridated and your child is going to the dentist for routine topical fluoride treatments, a fluoride dentifrice will give an added benefit. Study labels to choose a brand the American Dental Association's Council on Dental Therapeutics has tested and approved.

Fluorides in Mouthwashes

The new fluoride mouthwashes that are coming on the market today have been tested on school-age children, some of whom drank fluoridated wter and some of whom had only nonfluoridated water available. The results of the tests are impressive. If you decide to add a fluoride mouthwash to your home fluoride program, be sure to use it as directed, and see that your child uses it properly. Some types can be swallowed; others should not be.

Ways in Which You Can Get Fluoride to Your Child's Teeth

- Encouraging your child to drink water. All water contains some fluoride.
- Learning which foods contain fluoride, and making them part of the child's diet.
- Urging your community to bring the fluoride in its water supply up to optimum levels.
- Giving your child dietary supplements of fluoride in liquid or tablet form.
- Having your child brush with a fluoride dentifrice.
- Having your child rinse with a fluoride mouthwash after he brushes.
- Taking your child to the dentist's office for a regular checkup. The dentist will administer a topical fluoride treatment.

A MULTIPLE APPROACH

I think there's no doubt that a balanced multiple fluoride program will pay off for your child, and with very good reason. Under optimum conditions, a tooth comes into the mouth with about 800 ppm of fluoride in the outer layer of enamel. I'm talking about the teeth of a child whose drinking water contains 1 ppm of fluoride and whose teeth did not erupt unusually early, but remained in contact with the fluoride-bearing tissue fluids longer.

Now, this figure, 800 ppm, is not the optimum level for fluoride. Tests prove that levels of 1000 ppm and above are associated with caries resistance. Therefore, it is what we do after the teeth come in that can pull this level up. All the ways we use to bring fluoride in contact with the tooth are pushing that figure up the scale.

With all the talk about methods, costs, benefits, and statistics on fluoridation, let's not lose sight of the most interesting thing about fluoride: it works.

Caries Checklist

Preventive measures are a matter of routine for every day of the year. How does your family rate in the fight against decay?

- Does the baby get his or her teeth and gums wiped after feeding?
- Do the older children brush after meals to remove food and bacteria?
- Do you all clean once a day with brushing *and* flossing to break up plaque?
- Is your family getting fluoride?
- Are you eating too many refined, sweet foods?
- Do any members of the family snack between meals? What kinds of snacks are they — sweet and sticky or detergent? Do all of you at least clear your mouths with a swish-and-swallow?

SEVEN

A Visit to the Dentist

CHOOSING A DENTIST

There are a number of ways to find a dentist for your child. The most obvious ways are probably the best. First, you can ask your friends or other parents the name of the dentist who treats them or their children, and whether they like him. It is not always necessary to take your child to a dentist who specializes in dentistry for children. Indeed, in some parts of the country pedodontists are rare. (A pedodontist has spent from two to five years in postgraduate study, specializing in dental problems of children and the principles and techniques of child psychology. He is trained to handle all children, even those without special problems.)

It is important to find a dentist *who likes working with children.* There's an old saw in dentistry to the effect that there are more dentists afraid of children than there are children afraid of dentists. You want to find someone who is patient and considerate, someone who makes the time available so that your child can proceed to learn to accept dentistry at a reasonable rate of speed.

If none of your neighbors or playground or nursery school friends can recommend a dentist, ask your own family doctor or dentist for a professional recommendation. Tell him you are looking for a dentist who has a special ability for dealing with children. And don't compromise on the caliber of work. High-quality dentistry can, should be, and usually is done on children, with long-term benefits. If a dentist is not happy treating your child, just find another — dentist, that is. The only commodities a dentist has to sell are his time, his interest in your child, and his skill. He is not selling little bits of silver filling or x-ray film.

If the personal approach doesn't work or if you are new in your community, call the local dental health society. Most towns and cities have one. Ask for the names of dentists who like to work with children. You can also look in your local library for the American Dental Association's directory, which lists such specialties as pedodontics. Or you can telephone the nearest accredited hospital and ask the chief of dental service or the attending dentist to recommend several qualified dentists. In general, a personal recommendation is preferable.

The time to choose a dentist is before you need one. That way, you can take your time and make a reasoned, deliberate choice. You may want to pay a brief call on the dentist before a professional visit — even "interview" him — to explain that you are looking for a special kind of dentist and to ask him about his particular field and approach.

EVALUATING A DENTIST

I think you can expect the dentist and his staff to be familiar with dental disease, the techniques for identifying and removing plaque, the role of diet, eating habits, food substitutions, and the optimal use of systemic and topical fluorides. You might expect him to investigate and consider the application of sealants. And you'd expect skillful and painless repair, if it is needed, with the latest dental techniques and equipment.

After you've found your dentist, you'll be able to tell if he's interested in the growth and development of your child by noting whether he is concerned with filling teeth — cavity-oriented — or whether he deals with the prevention as well as the treatment of dental caries. A dentist should not be concerned just with repair work, and neither should you. This book should give you a broad knowledge of your child's teeth, not merely the ability to recognize danger signs. You'll be able to discern whether your dentist's orientation is toward the whole child.

MAKING HASTE SLOWLY

Making haste slowly is truly the best procedure for a child's first visit to the dentist. For example, when a three-year-old girl walks into my office for the first time, I ask her if she wants to climb up into the chair by herself (to lift her off her feet suddenly and without her approval could cause a terrific loss of her dignity). I sit; communication goes on at eye level. I speak in a low, calm voice — I don't need to produce any more excitement than is already present in the situation. I don't want to penetrate her personal space too rapidly, so I reach out — at arm's length — and take her hand. Counting her fingers (counting is a calm, prosaic procedure), I slowly draw closer to the chair. I think of the process as tell/show/do: I tell the child everything I am going to do, show her how I am going to do it, and then do exactly what I have said.

In the chair, my young patient is invited to look around, take a drink of water, and look at her teeth in a small hand mirror that she can hold herself while she and I count them. Watching what is going on is not only absorbing; it keeps her from imagining all sorts of things that are *not* going on.

We may discover some things that need help, which means that there may be repeated visits. If the child is very cooperative, I may take an x-ray or two on the first visit, but the more involved procedures are better left to later visits.

If we can just manage to talk and touch and understand each other a little bit, the two of us have really succeeded in doing a great deal on this first visit.

WHEN SHOULD THE FIRST VISIT TAKE PLACE?

I like to see a child for the first time when she is between two and three. By this time, all twenty primary teeth are in the mouth. Of course, if a younger child has cavities or has had an accident that injured the tooth, she will need to see a dentist even earlier.

HOW OFTEN SHOULD YOU RETURN
FOR A CHECKUP?

In general, dental visits should take place every six months, but that can vary. Some people are more susceptible to decay than others; some have better dental hygiene habits than others; some eat more sweets than others. Regular and frequent visits give the dentist an opportunity to discover problems *early,* which lowers the chances of the child's suffering pain, serious complications, and loss of teeth.

GETTING READY FOR THE FIRST VISIT

I know you feel you should prepare your child for her first visit to the dentist, but the less prepping you do, the better. Don't promise the child that the dentist will do anything more than look at her teeth. If the office is new to you, don't even try to describe what it will look like or what the office procedure will be. And don't discuss the dentist's equipment. You may use words that are not in the vocabulary of a dentist who treats children today. A pick or an explorer is a "tooth-feeler" in my office; a drill is a "tooth-cleaner"; fluoride solution is called a "tooth-shiner"; and words and phrases such as "hurt," "shot," "Novocain," "injections," "stick you with a needle" are not in my vocabulary. If I must do some work that will "bother" (not "hurt") the child, then I "put the tooth to sleep." Children, much to the surprise of most parents and many dentists, tolerate local anesthesia very well.

Let the child listen to the words the dentist uses and form her own impressions, experience her own sensations. She'll be better able to deal with it all.

Point one is to tell the child the truth. Don't exaggerate or embroider. Too often children who are brought to the dentist expect something entirely different from the experience that awaits them. Don't say, "This is not going to hurt," when there is no reason at all to set up and deal with the idea of pain before the child ever gets to the dentist's chair. Usually a first visit does not involve any procedure that will be uncomfortable. With today's modern techniques, including topical anesthesia, the dentist knows he's not going to hurt his patient. Should later treatment involve some discomfort, dentist and patient can get through it together if confidence has been built from the very first visit.

It's difficult for parents who have themselves had bad dental experiences to bring their children to the dentist without keying them in to their own fears. Children have very sensitive antennae.

Here's an old parent trick. You're taking your child to the dentist, and your own load of anxiety leads you to offer to buy her a toy, a comic book, or an ice-cream soda when the "visit" is over. The child knows something's up. Why would she be getting a treat in the middle of the afternoon? It's not even a special day. Or is it?

The parent's hand tightens. His voice gets a little higher. He grimaces, face muscles taut. The child is taking all this in.

I know it's difficult to hide your feelings. The best advice I have for a parent is that he try to believe that going to the dentist can be a nonthreatening, non-fear-provoking experience. It can even be a *good* experience — for parent, child, and dentist. Try to regard it as a *new* experience. You'll see your child relax and come into the office without carrying the burden of your apprehension.

SHOULD THE PARENT ACCOMPANY THE CHILD INTO THE TREATMENT ROOM?

The answer to this question depends on three people. Some parents do not have the ability to hand their children over to someone else's care, regardless of the confidence they may feel in the other person. The parent feels he has to protect, intervene, interpret.

The child may be comfortable in the unfamiliar environment of the dentist's office if he can see a familiar face. On the other hand, a child of even three or four may want Mommy there because she knows she can manipulate her by fussing or crying, but the dentist is an unknown quantity. It's not inconceivable that your four-year-old is taking the occasion to embarrass you, the parent who brought her here against her will.

If you panic at hearing your child cry in the treatment room, just stop and listen for a moment. Is this plain, everyday crying? Is it different from her crying when she wants to go skating or to have bedtime put off a little longer? Is it that special crying she has within her arsenal, her atom bomb? If it's familiar, treat it as you would under ordinary circumstances.

As for the dentist: some dentists are not comfortable with an audience, but prefer working and relating one-to-one with the child. And then some dentists are extroverts and enjoy performing their work in front of the parent and an assistant. Personality comes into it. Let the dentist make the decision. If he or she allows you to stay in the treatment room, remember that you are not a participant. Stay out of the child's vision — your expression and reaction may give a lot of wrong information to your observant child. No talking; no "This will be over in a minute," or "Wait till I tell Daddy how you behaved in the dentist's office." You are not there to applaud the child's good behavior or reprimand her when she doesn't cooperate. This is not three-way theater.

Personally, I'm more comfortable with the parent in the room, if he or she is a silent observer and sits behind the child so as not to provide facial or body cues. Sometimes it's most comforting for a preschooler to hold a parent's hand, and I have no objection to an infant or a very young child sitting in the parent's lap.

I've gone into all this to show you how certain methods work for me. I call them my "superstitions": the ways, procedures, and techniques that I find effective. I understand that it's a new experience for you, too; in fact, it's a triangle — child, parent, and dentist. If your dentist is comfortable working in different ways from those I describe, then he or she must do it his or her way, and will be equally successful.

Going to the dentist is not the same as going to a pediatrician, and parents shouldn't expect one experience to be translated into the other. The dentist is faced with different problems. First, he must have the child's cooperation. To do a proper cleaning, an accurate x-ray, a correct restoration, he needs the child's attention for, sometimes, fifteen to twenty minutes at a time. The pediatrician, who puts a child on a scale, looks in her throat, and listens to the chest, needs a shorter period of cooperation. For giving injections, a pediatrician may require only a few seconds to turn the child over, aim a needle, and let go; a dentist is searching for a tiny spot in the back of the jaw, with the tongue in the way . . .

Parents may find themselves helping their pediatrician by holding or supporting the child; they don't perceive the visit to the pediatrician as a threatening situation, and don't transmit tension to the child. Holding the child does not work in the dentist's office.

Another difference: often the child has to come to the dentist for a repeated number of visits, so the dentist must sustain the relationship from one visit to the next. Pediatric visits are generally separated by longer periods of time once the child is past infancy.

What do you do if you bring two children to the office — say, one three-year-old and one five-year-old? Do you put big brother in the chair and let the younger child watch?

Although it may surprise you — and perhaps your dentist — I'd advise letting the three-year-old go first. That's another one of my superstitions. If the three-year-old goes first and behaves well, the older child will feel that he must do as well. Also, the younger one has no way of interpreting what's being done to his big brother, so watching won't prepare him for his own experience. And he resents always being second banana.

I wouldn't worry about the effects of your child's crying on other children. Other children generally recognize crying for what it is: frustration, anger, manipulation.

If you are going to prepare the child for a first visit, follow the rule that applies to sex and politics: tell him no more than he's ready to hear. I myself would say something like this: "We're going to the dentist this afternoon. He's going to look at your teeth. When we get there you can sit in his special chair. He'll look in your mouth and count your teeth, and he'll tell you a little bit about how to take care of them."

Unfortunately, for some children that first visit is an emergency visit. The family has waited until a toothache came along. In that case, say: "A dentist is someone who takes care of your teeth when they hurt and fixes them so they can get better. That's why we're going to the dentist."

As with any new subject, answer only the questions your child asks, giving him or her information on the appropriate level, and no more than he or she wants to know at that time. And when you don't know something, admit it — don't make up an answer.

X-RAY EXAMINATIONS

The x-ray is a valuable diagnostic tool for the dentist. Decay can proceed so rapidly in children that it is important to detect a cavity as soon as possible. Cavities still too small to be seen by the naked eye will show up on an x-ray. And decay spots between the teeth, where a mirror and explorer can't reach, can be located by x-ray.

Extra teeth, missing teeth — any anomaly in the permanent teeth, which are still buried in the jaw — can be seen on x-rays. This information is needed if the dentist must decide whether to retain or remove teeth.

Parents, dentists, and physicians are justifiably concerned about the proliferating and extensive use of x-rays. There is incontrovertible evidence that people who receive excessive x-ray therapy as children develop problems, especially malignancies of soft tissues, in later life. Excessive use of x-rays should be avoided whenever possible.

Today's machines are safe and easily operated. When I finished dental school, an x-ray took one or one and one-half seconds of exposure time. Today, new, shielded equipment takes x-rays in tenths of a second; fifteen or twenty pictures can be taken in the time it took for one of the old-style exposures. The amount of radiation a child gets from once-a-year x-rays is less than he'd get from natural sources during a day at the beach. And in my office a child who has good six-month reports doesn't get an x-ray at every visit.

X-ray machines that can take a single panoramic picture of the jaws are already in use. The subject sits still, and the film, in a flexible cassette, is placed on a rotating drum. It shifts around and takes a full shot of all primary and permanent teeth. This, with a few cavity-checking pictures, should be enough for the dentist's diagnostic needs.

ANESTHESIA

There may be times when a young child — a preschooler, perhaps — has to have extensive dentistry done (maybe oral surgery) and the dentist will suggest general anesthesia so that he can control the child during the work that must be done.

General Anesthesia

I think all parents should be aware that general anesthesia used on a young child entails a great deal of risk. A child who loses consciousness under general anesthesia loses his protective reflexes. Because of his small body size, he carries a smaller amount of oxygen in his lungs than does an adult. For him there are risks an adult — or even a nine- or ten-year-old — does not face.

I believe you should ask the dentist this question: "Can somebody else perform the work under local anesthesia?"

It may be worth seeking a specialist who works just with children. He has the training in psychology and in the treatment of very young children that may make it possible for him to do the work under local anesthesia. Tragedies do occur under general anesthesia. If I must use it — and there are several times a year when I have no choice but to do so — my strong opinion is that dentistry performed on a child under general anesthesia should be done in a hospital, where the anesthesia is administered by an anesthesiologist — a physician who specializes in this field. This reduces risk. If I can, I arrange to have a pediatric anesthesiologist assist me. He concentrates on anesthetic management and I am free to do my work.

Local Anesthesia

Most adults have grown up with a fear of needles and injections. Today, with the development of new wire needles and new topical anesthetics, it is entirely possible to give a child an injection so that she feels nothing more than a slight pulling sensation.

Dentists are trained to administer local anesthetics, and can do so with skill. The psychological preparation of dentist and child is important.

EIGHT

Orthodontics

What I am going to say here will sound controversial to some orthodontists and confusing to some parents, but when you think about
it, it's logical.

WHEN IS ORTHODONTICS NEEDED?

By and large, most people seek orthodontic treatment because the
teeth don't look good. Appearance is what motivates an individual
to seek orthodontic therapy.

It is a strong, valid reason.

We live in a world where a bright smile and straight, even teeth
contribute to social and professional success. The lack of such a smile
leads to self-consciousness and misery. Most parents do not want
their child to be handicapped by an unattractive appearance.

Some people think that teeth that are straight, well-spaced, well-
aligned, and lacking an overbite are healthy teeth. Not necessarily.
They're just pretty. For the most part, crooked teeth are not inher-
ently unhealthy teeth. A couple of rotated teeth in the front of the
mouth might create a cleaning problem, but in general, spaces, leaning teeth, and crookedness are neither dangerous nor unhealthy.

There are some rare instances where orthodontics becomes medi-
cally necessary. Examples of these are inherited disorders, such as
infantile osteomyelitis, a chronic infection of the bones; accidents
and injuries; and a form of ankylosis (abnormal bone fusion) in

which partially unerupted permanent teeth become fused with the jawbone and stop short of arriving fully in the mouth. But these rare conditions are just that — rare — and you'll be aware of them as such.

If I were a parent making a decision about orthodontics for my child, I would first decide that I did not like the appearance of the permanent teeth, and then find out whether the child feels the same way. If you both feel strongly that the appearance is unsightly, then it is reasonable to choose orthodonture.

OCCLUSION

There is no absolute standard for the way teeth fit or look, and it is not necessary to search for one. As a matter of fact, such a search would probably end in a look of "falseness" — standardization — whereas most teeth have as much individuality as their owners.

Occlusion — the way the teeth fit together when the jaw is closed — is also different in each person. Occlusion changes throughout a person's life — as baby teeth are shed, adult teeth arrive, growth patterns change, and wear and habit accomplish their effects.

When occlusion is good, both sides of the jaw and face are matching, or symmetrical. You would probably notice a sideward swing of the lower jaw, a sign of malocclusion, which is discussed below. If you want to look at your child's teeth in occlusion, instead of asking him to "open up," ask him to show you his mouth with his lips open and his teeth closed.

Notice that the front teeth project ahead of their matching bottom teeth. That's called "overjet." The top teeth also extend down, covering their matching lower teeth to some degree. That is called "overbite." These are normal conditions. Don't try to diagnose malocclusion on the basis of your own judgment or impressions. It is a relative thing, and whatever your opinions may be, you will need the advice of a person specially trained and experienced in the dental and facial development of the child.

It's quite a surprise to parents when the small, neat, white baby teeth are lost and the enormous, ivory permanent teeth erupt. After all, these are fully grown adult teeth coming into a jaw and face that still belong to a child. Especially during the months of mixed dentition, when your child shows a mixture of baby teeth, adult teeth, and gaps, you may wonder if you'll ever get used to his new look. This is a perfectly natural effect; it's temporary; and it is no sign of malocclusion.

MALOCCLUSION

Any deviation from the normal way in which the teeth of the upper jaw meet and fit with the teeth of the lower jaw is called malocclusion.

Malocclusion can result in problems:

- When teeth don't meet properly, they cannot perform their regular cutting and grinding action. This sometimes leads to the person's avoiding foods needed in a balanced and varied diet because they are just too difficult to eat.
- There may be displacement of the lower jaw in relation to the upper jaw, with resulting lack of symmetry, pressure on the anterior portion of the ear, pain in the mandibular jaw hinge.
- Distress about appearance may arise.

CHOOSING AN ORTHODONTIST

Choosing an orthodontist is a big step. Like plastic surgery, it's done only once, and the esthetic result is one that the child will have to live with throughout her life. In financial terms, it's like buying a car; it's expensive.

Most orthodontists will take a series of x-rays and make study casts of the child's mouth in preparing a treatment plan. If you want another opinion as to the mode of treatment or cost or anything else, don't be embarrassed to ask the orthodontist to send his records to another dentist for his or her opinion. It's done all the time. I myself am quite pleased to send my records to someone else for evaluation. To me, such a request means that the parents are involved, interested, and aware of what is happening. This always leads to better treatment for the child.

Some cautions:

- Don't be upset if the second orthodontist chooses a different course of treatment. There are many different appliances and ways of achieving a healthy, esthetic result. In asking for another opinion, you always run the risk of confusing yourself. If this should happen, continue to ask questions until you and your child feel comfortable with the answers. Fortunately, when it comes to orthodontics, there are no emergencies.

- Don't expect the orthodontist to give the study casts and x-rays to you. Surprisingly, the law says that they belong to him. However, it is customary and proper for him to send them to another orthodontist for an opinion should you request it.

- An orthodontist usually won't be able to tell you exactly how long treatment will take. Each child is a separate psychological and biological entity. In orthodontics, cooperation from the child is important. Without it, treatment takes many extra months. Children grow at different rates, and no one can predict how much growth will occur during any course of treatment.

PREVENTIVE ORTHODONTICS

The general dental practitioner or the pedodontist who has been seeing your child in the early years can and does practice preventive orthodontics. He tries to prevent the premature loss of primary teeth due to decay or accident; saves room for adult teeth when primary teeth are prematurely lost; repairs primary teeth, when necessary, accurately and carefully to maintain the tooth's shape and function. These things are effective in an orthodontic dimension, too.

For example, suppose a primary tooth is lost before it should be — perhaps knocked out in a fall. Your dentist may recommend the use of a temporary space maintainer. This is a metal device that will hold the space open until the permanent tooth is ready to grow into its proper position. A similar device sometimes is used to regain space already lost.

Maintaining the space, however, is not always necessary. In the front of the mouth, space seems to stabilize. If a space maintainer is needed anywhere, it is usually in the back of the mouth. It is important to keep the appropriate relationships in the back teeth, but even here, a space maintainer is not always needed.

What can happen if the space is not saved when it should be? The teeth on each side may begin to tip over into the space. The matching tooth in the opposite jaw, meeting no resistance, will grow longer. Drifting teeth cause the stresses of chewing to be distributed unevenly, which is not good for the supporting bones and gums. It's a situation that may call, in a few years, for a full set of braces.

It's just as important to keep watch for teeth that are retained too long. When primary teeth stay around after they should be gone, they leave the incoming permanent teeth with nowhere to go but sideways. If you have made a practice of counting your child's teeth and becoming familiar with his mouth, you yourself will become aware that a baby tooth has been around longer than it should be.

As I have said, when a tooth comes into the mouth, it doesn't know where it's going. It follows the path of least resistance, and responds to the environment it finds itself in. Among the most important environmental factors determining the position of the permanent teeth are bad mouth habits, such as thrusting one's tongue against the upper teeth with each swallow, biting one's lower lip, thus pushing the upper teeth out and the lower teeth in, and thumbsucking. After the child is six, when the permanent teeth begin to come in, these habits begin to cause problems.

Here are two very important questions to ask the orthodondist: "Is my child's malocclusion due to a bad habit?" "Will the habit still be there after the work is done?"

The preventive dentistry that deals with troublesome habits is called "interceptive dentistry." If a developing orthodontic problem can be intercepted, many malocclusions can be prevented entirely, or treatment can be greatly reduced. It may be as simple as controlling

an incipient crossbite in an erupting incisor with an exercise performed with a wooden tongue depressor.

Your regular dentist or pedodontist can advise you if and when
you need to consult an orthodontist.

HOW ORTHODONTICS WORKS

Attaining normal occlusion is the job of the pediatric dentist. Regain-
ing normal occlusion is the job of the orthodontist. Orthodontics is
the branch of dentistry that specializes in attaining normal occlusion
for the patient. It includes both preventive and corrective measures.
An orthodontist has had postgraduate work in this specialty.

The physiological basis for orthodontics is the fact that bone is not
hard and unyielding, as we generally think of it. Bone is flexible and
malleable. The orthodontist, by applying long-term gentle pressure
with various appliances and through exercises, can slowly bring teeth
back into occlusion. Bone yields to the pressure in front of the tooth,
and new bone forms and hardens behind it.

The kinds of appliances and materials used in orthodontics have
not changed very much over the years: springs, wires, rubber bands,
braces with plastic or metal brackets, some attached and some removable. What has changed more than methods and materials is the
timing. Dentists are recognizing beginning malocclusions and treating them early. In fact, many dentists now believe that much expensive and lengthy orthodontic treatment in the teen years can be
avoided by recognizing and treating occlusion problems when the
child is as young as four or five.

HOW LONG SHOULD IT TAKE?

If too much pressure is applied when a tooth is moved through bone
with an appliance, the root of the tooth may be resorbed instead of
the bone that the tooth is supposed to move through. In other words,
too much pressure from the appliance can loosen a tooth — even

extract it! The orthodontist must put just the right pressure on the tooth to move it without letting the root be lost. That's why you may have to expect two and a half or perhaps even three and a half years for orthodontics to be completed. There is no set schedule. Everybody is different, and every orthodontic problem is different. Patient cooperation can shorten markedly the time of treatment.

HOW MUCH SHOULD IT COST?

Many parents wonder why orthodontics is so expensive. Orthodontic treatment takes a great deal of planning by the dentist before the braces go on. And a great deal of time must be spent in making adjustments. It is not uncommon for a child to visit the orthodontist for half an hour every two weeks. Over a period of three years, this really adds up.

HOW MUCH SHOULD IT HURT?

Orthodontics should be painless. If the teeth feel sore for several days after an adjustment, tell your orthodontist; the braces are too tight.

If a wire or band is irritating or cutting the tissue of the mouth, the parent or child can apply a little bit of first-aid with a piece of soft wax or sugarless chewing gum. Smooth it over the edge to make things more comfortable until the orthodontist can correct the problem.

Removable or Fixed Appliances?

The question of whether removable or fixed appliances should be used has to be decided by the dentist. Removable appliances are generally used for minor or short-term corrections (six months to a year).

For major, long-term work, the fixed appliance gives the dentist more control. Success doesn't depend on the child's remembering to wear it. No matter how careful everyone promises to be, removable appliances are always getting lost at the bottom of a swimming pool or getting sat on in someone's back pocket. The need for constant repair or replacement is expensive and is an irritation for the child and a pain for the dentist.

By the way, there are now white — tooth-colored — brackets that bond onto teeth, and they are not unsightly. Not that braces are much of a problem anymore. Wearing them has become "in"; it's a sign of self-esteem, which children display with a certain nonchalance. Nowadays much orthodontics is done before the self-conscious teen years.

ORAL HYGIENE DURING ORTHODONTICS

Orthodontics is dangerous for somebody who has a high caries history. The reason is that the child does not clean his teeth terribly well in the first place. Dental caries, as noted before, is a multifactorial disease. Bands and braces may be just that extra factor that weights the balance on the negative side.

Every child in orthodontics should realize that he will have to make an extra effort to keep his mouth clean. It is heartbreaking to have a child enter orthodontic treatment with no cavities, and then find, when the bands and braces are removed, nice straight teeth full of decay. While the child is undergoing orthodontics may be the time for a water-irrigating device to be added to your cleaning equipment.

NINE

Prevention Today

BACKGROUND OF THE
PREVENTIVE DENTISTRY MOVEMENT

In the late 1960s and early 1970s, there was a great and enthusiastic movement throughout the United States among dentists and in schools and health education programs for something called "preventive dentistry." The control of dental disease seemed within our grasp; it was an exciting time.

What triggered this movement was exact information from laboratories in scientific fields as diverse as physical chemistry, oral microbiology, and nutritional biochemistry. For the first time, we knew exactly what happens in the formation of dental caries. We thought we had known for a long time, but now we had clinical proof.

Many of us were encouraged to think that if we could eliminate the dental plaque that makes caries possible, we could eliminate dental disease for all time! Dentists, parents, and teachers all mounted an attack on plaque. The focus of this effort was the identification of plaque by the use of disclosing solutions, and then its removal by brushing and flossing.

The problem is that, although theoretically one can prevent the formation of caries by a program of vigorous brushing and flossing twice a day, one cannot make people stick to such a program. For too many people, children and adults alike, the personal effort just doesn't become a routine, like combing your hair or tying your shoelaces. Even dental students, who were given the opportunity and were encouraged to follow a careful regimen, still got plaque on their teeth. And even they had difficulty removing it completely.

The situation is not so different from two other health concerns. People know that neither cigarettes nor high cholesterol diets without proper exercise are good for them. But how many make the effort to change the way they live? If doctors can't get people to stop smoking, if they can't get them to eat wisely and exercise, how are they going to get them to brush and floss regularly? Just telling people what is good for them is not enough.

I was not the only one to become discouraged. Many people lost confidence in the preventive dentistry movement as an effective means of ending dental caries for the population as a whole. Theoretically, it's possible; practically, it doesn't work.

I have not the slightest doubt that I can take a highly motivated child with a highly motivated parent and get them started on a program of tooth care that results in immaculate teeth for a period of time. Then the question — the real question — arises: Will they still be so careful two, three, six months from now?

The answer is no.

What happens is that the commitment just doesn't hold up. Yes, there are dentists who can make it work. A dentist can spend all his time constantly urging and supervising his patients in the practice of preventive dentistry. An unusual relationship like that might work, but it entails such dependency and such involvement between dentist and patient that it is impractical and unrealistic. I don't think a patient should become wedded to his dentist.

My father is a dentist, a devoted practitioner of preventive dentistry. He still believes that it's the way to prevent dental disease. I don't. I believe the best we can hope for is to *improve* the brushing and flossing habits of as many people as possible. We can give people the tools and the information. Then the use of these tools and information is something they must practice on their own.

The Defensive Program at My House

- My children brush twice, floss once a day. My wife and I check at least once daily to make sure all plaque is gone.
- They use a fluoride dentifrice.
- They rinse with a fluoride mouthwash once a day.
- They don't get sugar snacks. (Actually, they're not even interested because they've never had the opportunity to develop a taste for chocolates and other sweets.)
- Twice a year they get a checkup that includes prophylaxis (cleaning) and a topical fluoride treatment.
- They use plaque-disclosing tablets about once a week as a self-check to see how good a cleaning job they are doing.

DEFENSIVE TOOLS

These are the best defensive tools anybody has today:

1. *Vigorous toothbrushing and daily flossing.* These procedures should be utilized at least once every 24 hours to disrupt the formation of plaque.
2. *Fluoride in the water supply.* There is no question in my mind or anybody else's that if one child grows up in a neighborhood with a fluoridated water supply, and another has access only to nonfluoridated water, by the time the children are in high school, the one without fluoridated water will have about 50 percent more dental cavities than the other. That's a persuasive statistic.
3. *A Good Diet.* I know very well that your child is not going to give up sweets and sticky snacks, no matter how strongly I condemn them. But if you can understand how sugar causes dental decay, you can begin to control when and how much of these foods he eats.

This is a defensive dental program. It can work for your family. It can make your children members of a cavity-free generation. The real day-to-day battle is the battle against decay. This is one war you don't want to lose; a caries-destroyed tooth, unlike a broken bone, can never repair or regenerate itself.

THE NUMBERS GAME

I know that statistics are dull, and I've tried to avoid them. But statistics have a message, so let's take a look at these:

- Half of all two-year-olds have one or more cavities.
- Half the children in the United States under the age of fifteen have never received any dental care.
- If you are over six years of age, chances are 8 out of 10 that you have several cavities in your mouth.
- If you are twenty, you have fourteen decayed, missing, or filled teeth.
- If you are sixty, chances are 9 in 10 that you don't have a tooth in your head!

Here's another way of putting this: 111 million adult Americans have 2.25 billion decayed, missing, or filled teeth.

These are all different statistical ways of saying that nobody paid very much attention to preventive dentistry until a few years ago. And even today, when control of dental disease is within our grasp, up to 98 percent of all children will, at some time in their school lives, experience tooth decay.

Old Wives' Tale

"Losing teeth is just part of getting old — like gray hair and wrinkles. Sooner or later, everybody wears dentures."
Nonsense. Teeth were designed to last as long as you do. With proper care, at home and at the dentist's, you can keep your teeth for a lifetime, a long one.

That the efforts of dental education have had some effect seems borne out by recent statistics. Before the middle of the century, most people went to the dentist for extractions, fillings, and dentures. Today, the percentage of people going to the dentist for checkups, cleaning, x-rays, and surface amalgam fillings — services we can describe as preventive — is constantly increasing.

Fluoride treatments	454% increase
Root canal therapies	124% increase
Orthodontic sittings	127% increase
Extractions	6.7% decrease
Periodontal treatments	0.7% decrease
Fillings and inlays	0.1% decrease

Of course, as more people go to the dentist for cleaning, x-ray examination, fluoride treatment, and orthodontic corrections, fewer will have to go for radical treatment. The swing of the tide is very slow, as the statistics show.

DENTISTRY OF THE FUTURE

Research on several fronts is turning up new technologies for the dentistry of the future. For example, there are new restorative materials — space-age materials — that can repair a tooth that used to be a candidate for a cap. A crack in a tooth can be glued over, and an unusually wide gap between teeth — between front incisors, for instance — can be closed by building up the sides of the separated teeth with new materials.

A novel approach that promises to turn us into a nation of music lovers is exercise programs designed to prevent crooked teeth by encouraging us to use certain musical instruments, such as sousaphones and trumpets. There are also exercises with buttons and other devices that may reduce the need for orthodontics.

More future "possibles" are listed below. A vast amount of research on these and other solutions to dental problems is going on at this moment. Meanwhile, keep brushing and flossing.

Miracles Coming Up (But Don't Hold Your Breath)

- A chemical that can remove tooth decay and plaque.
- An enzyme that will knock out decay-causing bacteria in the mouth.
- A plaque-removing dentifrice.
- A dentifrice that will remove stains *and* will strengthen gums.
- A vaccine against gum disease and cavities.
- A sealant for the entire tooth. (Sealants for tooth surfaces are already past the experimental stage.)
- A fluoride disk, cemented onto a back molar, that will allow time-release of fluoride in proper amounts.
- An additive to breakfast cereals that inhibits decay.
- Implantation of healthy bacteria that, thriving, will crowd out the bad guys. (There's room for only so many.)
- Electrical anesthesia. (An electric current depolarizes the pain nerve in the tooth — a truly painless drill.)
- Salivary analysis that will predict whether you will, or will not, be a caries-former.
- No-pain needles: fine, thin, disposable needles that don't occasion even an "ouch!"
- Ultrasonic drills that work superfast.
- Ultrasonic cleaning methods that will shake the tartar right off the teeth.
- Colorless orthodontic appliances.
- New transplant methods. (You may wind up wearing somebody else's tooth.)
- New filling materials that match tooth color, even for fillings in back teeth.
- Fiberoptic techniques that will give an instant analysis of the condition of your mouth, doing away with the need for x-rays.
- Carbon implants for roots of missing teeth.

Index

Thumb-sucking habit, 3, 13, 14,
129
Tongue-thrusting habit, 13, 40–41,
129
Tongue-tie, 24
Toothache, 74
emergency treatment, 75–76
Toothbrushes, 36, 50–51
electric, 51, 88
Toothbrushing, 50–53, 83
buddy system, 95
Tooth enamel, 4, 10
Tooth fairy, 57

Tooth-grinding habit, 42–
43

Vitamins, 4, 5, 71
fluoride with, 108

Water-irrigating devices, 52–53,
88–89
Water Pik, 52
Wisdom teeth, 53, 64
X-rays
during pregnancy, 7
examinations, 122–23